Nummular - shape of stacked coins
guttate - shape of a drop

W9-CZS-624

DIAGNOSTIC PICTURE TESTS IN

RHEUMATOLOGY

mycosis - relating to fungus
hyperkeratosis - excess Thicking of horny layer

V. Wright MD, FRCP
ARC Professor of Rheumatology
University of Leeds
Leeds, England

A. R. Harvey MRCP
Senior Registrar in Rheumatology
Rheumatism Research Unit
University of Leeds, England

YEAR BOOK MEDICAL PUBLISHERS, INC.

Titles in this series, published or being developed, include:

Diagnostic Picture Tests in Pediatrics

Picture Tests in Human Anatomy

Diagnostic Picture Tests in Oral Medicine

Diagnostic Picture Tests in Orthopedics

Diagnostic Picture Tests in Infectious Diseases

Diagnostic Picture Tests in Dermatology

Diagnostic Picture Tests in Ophthalmology

Diagnostic Picture Tests in Rheumatology

Diagnostic Picture Tests in Obstetrics/Gynecology

Diagnostic Picture Tests in Neurology

Diagnostic Picture Tests in Sports Injuries

Picture Tests in Surgical Diagnosis

Copyright © V. Wright & A. Harvey, 1987
Published by Wolfe Medical Publications Ltd, 1987
Printed by W. S. Cowell Ltd, Ipswich, England

Library of Congress Cataloging in Publication Data
Wright, Verna.
    Diagnostic picture tests in rheumatology.
    1. Rheumatism—Diagnosis—Examinations, questions, etc. 2. Arthritis—
Diagnosis—Examinations, questions, etc, 3. Rheumatism—Diagnosis—Atlases.
4. Arthritis—Diagnosis—Atlases. I. Harvey, Andrew R. II. Title.
[DNLM: 1. Rheumatism—diagnosis—atlases. 2. Rheumatism—diagnosis—
examination questions. WE 18 W953d]
RC927.W75 1987   616.7′23075′076   86–23390
ISBN 0 8151 9358 0

Preface

One of the major changes in medicine has been the recognition that rheumatological disorders have a far larger place in general medicine than the locomotor system alone. All organs of the body can be affected by rheumatic disorders and research activities in this discipline include the study of immunology, cellular biology, the haemostatic system and mineral metabolism as well as clinical pharmacology and therapeutics.

Professor Wright and Dr Harvey have made a significant contribution to both undergraduate and postgraduate teaching in this fine book. They have presented many diagnostic problems, clinical photographs and X-rays which provide the stimulation and self-motivation essential for effective learning. I have no doubt that this type of instruction forms an essential part of the learning process as the reader positively tests his knowledge. The quality and range of the illustrations are impressive, presenting an image to the mind which powerfully reinforces both learning and memory.

I wish that this type of book had been available when I was a student. If learning can become stimulating in this way it is doubly valuable, encouraging students to learn more and also retain their knowledge.

Professor C.R.M. Prentice
Head of Department of Medicine,
University of Leeds

Acknowledgements

Much co-operation is needed to collect 200 photographs which illustrate a specialist subject comprehensively. We would like to thank the following colleagues for their generous help in locating specific pictures and for giving permission to use their slides and photographs of patients:

Dr B M Ansell
Dr H A Bird
Dr W P Butt
Dr M A Chamberlain
Dr J A Cotterill
Dr A M Denman
Dr G J Hardy
Mr J S Hillman

Dr J M Iveson
Dr M R Jeffrey
Dr M F R Martin
Mr B A Noble
Dr H Pullen
Mr B Statham
Mr K S Taylor

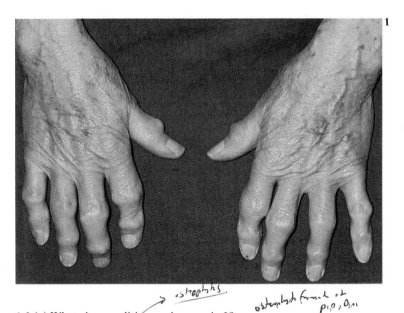

1,2 (a) What abnormalities can be seen in **2**?

(b) What are the swellings over the fingers in **1**? What do they consist of?

(c) What is the diagnosis? What features differentiate this from rheumatoid arthritis?

[handwritten annotations: osteophytes; osteophyte formation at PIP, DIP; OA; PIP, DIP involvement, no systemic involvement; osteoporosis / Thumbs; 1) stiffness relieved by a few minutes; 2) ↓ inflammation; 3) no systemic involvement]

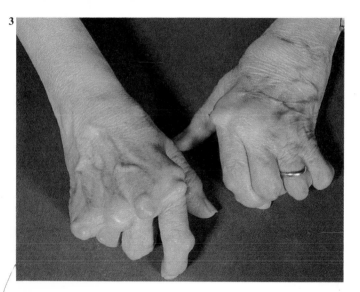

3 (a) What three diagnostic features can be seen in these arthritic hands?
(b) In what other anatomical locations may the skin signs be observed?
(c) At what single visceral site are these lesions most likely to cause diagnostic confusion?
(d) The patient developed septic arthritis of the elbow. What was the association with the skin abnormality?

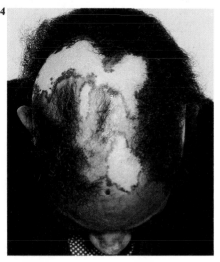

4 (a) What abnormalities are shown?
(b) What connective tissue disease is probable here?

Systemic Lupus: Erythematosis
inflammatory connective tiss. disorder
visible swelling including
fatigue, weakness, joint pain
lung fibrosis, skin disorder rash Reddish
pleurisy, + disease blood / kidney
lymphadenopathy, pericarditis
anaemia, hyperglobulinaemia
positive LE cell test

5 A 58-year-old man has a 20-year history of arthropathy affecting the feet and hands.
(a) What abnormalities can be seen?
(b) What is the diagnosis?
(c) After starting specific treatment, the patient developed urinary calculi. What type of treatment was given? What investigation might have given warning of this potential complication?
(d) What alternative drug should be used? What precaution should be taken following commencement of this drug?

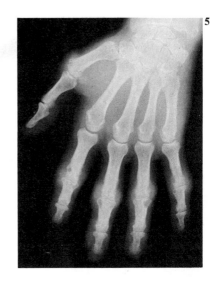

6 A woman with nodular rheumatoid arthritis complained of profound lethargy and progressive ankle oedema.
(a) What is the probable cause of this clinical sign, and how would you investigate further?
(b) What management should be considered?

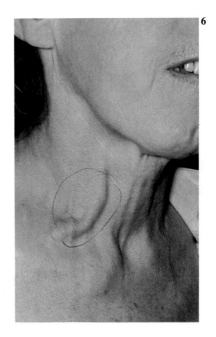

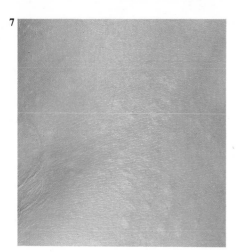

7,8 A skin abnormality was observed on the sides of the neck and axillae of a young man with joint hypermobility.
(a) What is the diagnosis?
(b) What is shown by the retinal photograph?
(c) What other clinical manifestations may this condition present? With what systemic rheumatological condition may it therefore be confused?
(d) What is the inheritance of this condition?

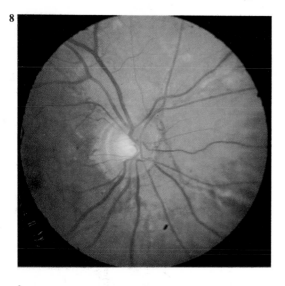

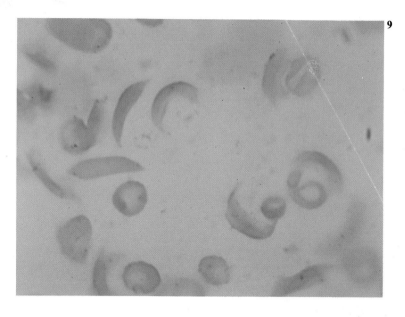

9 (a) What abnormality is shown in this bone marrow smear?
(b) What should be the primary concern in a patient with this condition presenting with bone or joint pain? Which specific causative factor is often implicated?
(c) Name four other mechanisms of bone or joint pain?

10 (a) A patient has ankylosing spondylitis. What test should be used to quantify the sign demonstrated for sequential monitoring?
(b) What other measures of skeletal mobility are useful in monitoring this condition?

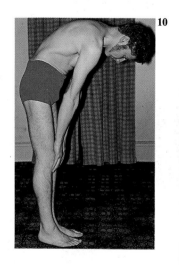

(hyperkeratotic scaly skin lesions)

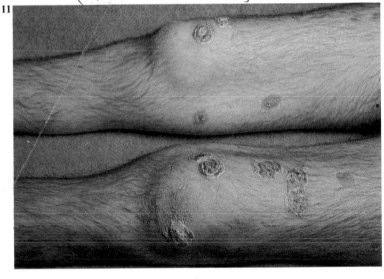

11,12 (a) Describe the skin lesions?

(b) What two diagnoses should be considered for these patients, who both have a relatively short history of skin abnormality and joint pain?

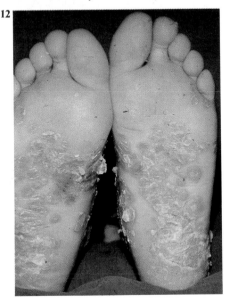

(c) What rheumatological features do these two conditions also have in common?

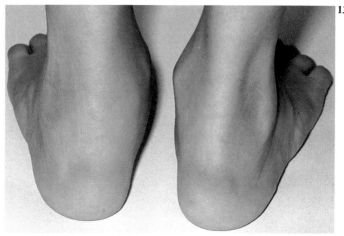

13 A teenage boy presented with heel and ankle pain. He remembered falling awkwardly 2 weeks previously.
(a) What can be observed?
(b) He had previously had dandruff, and showed an abnormality of the scalp and finger- and toe-nails. What is the probable diagnosis?

14 An oblique lumbar spinal X-ray of a 23-year-old competitive gymnast with back pain.
(a) What abnormality is shown? What is the probable cause?
(b) Into which four aetiological groups can the deformity associated with this condition be classified?
(c) What is the most serious potential complication? In which group is this most likely?

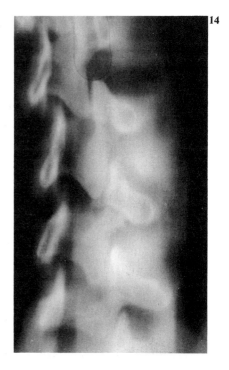

15

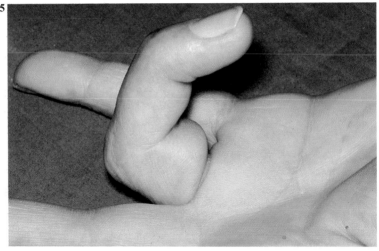

15 A young musician's ring finger occasionally became stuck in flexion. Extension of the finger was painful.
(a) What is this condition? What is the underlying abnormality?
(b) What is the probable cause? How should this patient be managed?

16

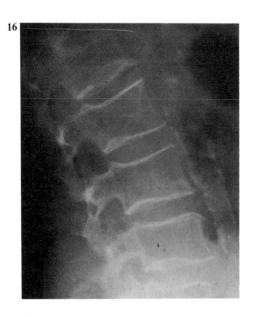

16 An elderly woman presented with sudden exacerbation of chronic back pain.
(a) What is the probable cause of the acute pain?
(b) What underlying abnormality is probable?
(c) What drug treatments have been shown to slow the progression of this condition?

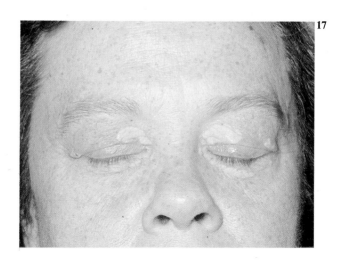

17 A 55-year-old woman presented with periodic symmetrical pain of the hands and feet of inflammatory type. Examination did not show objective joint signs, but nodules were present over the knuckles.
(a) What does the photograph show? What is the probable nature of the knuckle nodules? With what subtypes of this disorder may these clinical features be associated?
(b) What radiographic features may be seen at affected joints?
(c) What treatment should be advised for the joint symptoms and the underlying condition?

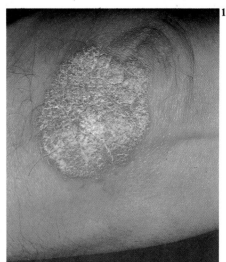

18 (a) What is the skin lesion on this elbow, which may be associated with arthropathy?
(b) What other less obvious sites for this condition should be examined?

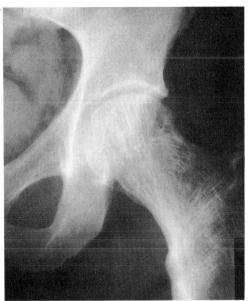

19–21 A 60-year-old man with established bone disease presented with a warm, painful, enlarging swelling at the right lower humerus.

(a) What is the bone disorder shown in the femur?

(b) What complication has occurred in the humerus, and what characteristic radiographic features are present?

(c) What therapy is indicated? What is the prognosis?

20

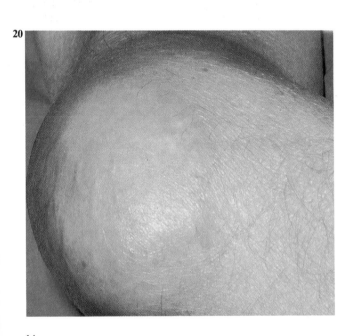

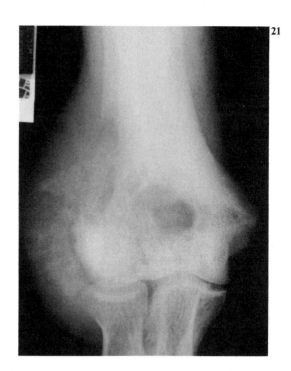

22 A 19-year-old woman presented with an acute painful swelling of the left knee, and fever.
(a) What additional abnormality is illustrated?
(b) What is the diagnosis?
(c) How could the diagnosis be confirmed?

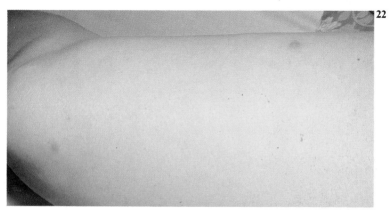

23 A 35-year-old woman with rheumatoid arthritis became progressively troubled by pain and tightness behind the left knee.
(a) What abnormality is shown?
(b) What relatively common complication of this condition may cause diagnostic difficulty in general practice, and why?
(c) What is the most useful investigation if diagnostic difficulty arises?

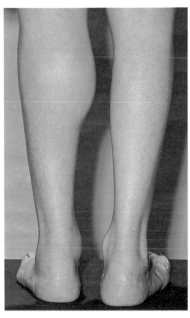

24 (a) What is the most prominent feature shown? What is the probable underlying diagnosis?
(b) What complication may result? How may it be prevented?

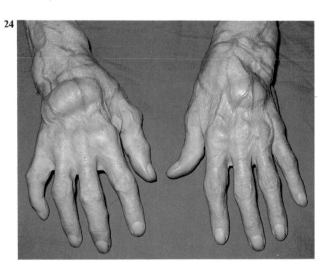

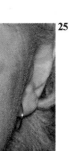

25 A patient experienced gradual stiffening of the fingers and tightness of the facial skin over several years.
(a) What skin abnormality is shown? What is the diagnosis?
(b) At what other site may similar skin abnormalities help to make this diagnosis?
(c) What relationship has been proposed between these skin changes and the pathogenesis of this condition?

26 (a) What is the probable cause of these chest X-ray abnormalities in a patient with systemic lupus erythematosus?
(b) What two other causes must be considered?
(c) What is the commonest respiratory abnormality in SLE?
(d) Asymptomatic lung function abnormality may be present in this condition. What specific investigations should be requested?

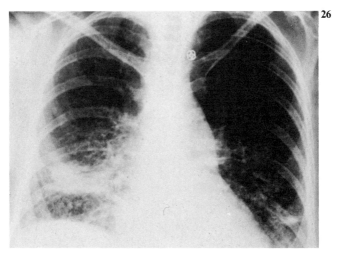

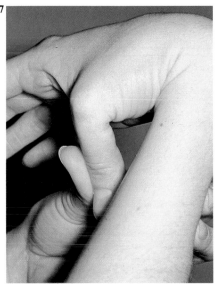

27,28 (a) What is being demonstrated?
(b) Of which inherited disorders may this be a feature?
(c) With what rheumatological complaints may simple hypermobility present?
(d) At what age do symptoms usually commence?
(e) How can joint hypermobility be simply quantitated?

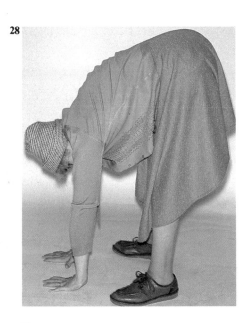

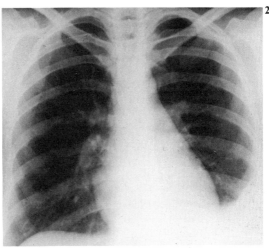

29 This X-ray demonstrates the commonest respiratory complication of rheumatoid disease.
(a) How would this be expected to present?
(b) What is the sex-incidence of this complication?
(c) What differential diagnosis should be considered? Does the fluid have any diagnostic features?

30 A woman with rheumatoid arthritis complained of recent exacerbation of hand pain, particularly troublesome at night.
(a) What relevant abnormalities are shown?
(b) What is the probable cause of her hand pain? How could this be investigated?
(c) What three possible forms of treatment should be considered?

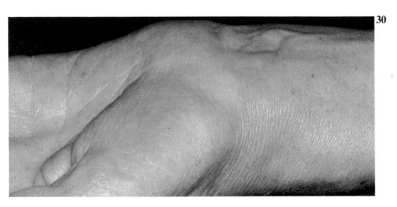

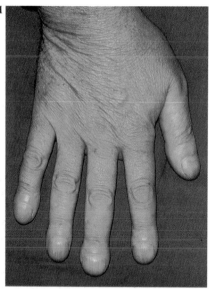

31 A 67-year-old man presented with hand, wrist and ankle pain and swelling, and weight loss.

(a) What sign is shown in this hand photograph?

(b) What is the clinical syndrome described? What are the causes?

(c) What surgical treatments may dramatically improve this condition?

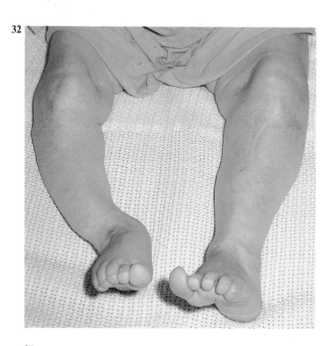

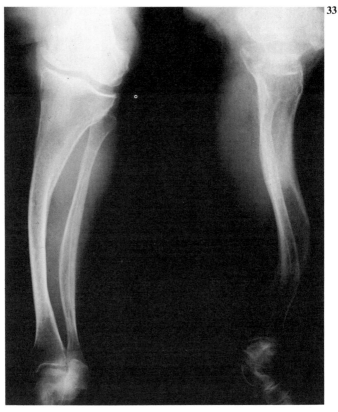

32,33 A short-statured patient complained of knee pain.
(a) What is the cause of the knee pain?
(b) What is the cause of the abnormal bone shape?

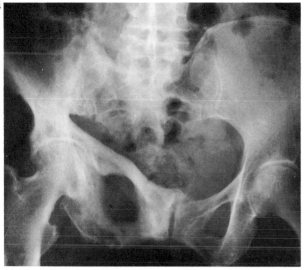

34 (a) To what can this pelvic deformity be attributed?
(b) What secondary complication has occurred?
(c) What surgical problems might be posed by right hip replacement?

35 This uncommon skin manifestation may complicate ulcerative colitis and rheumatoid arthritis.
(a) What is it?
(b) What are the characteristic clinical features?
(c) What is the probable pathogenesis?

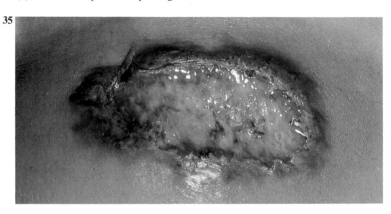

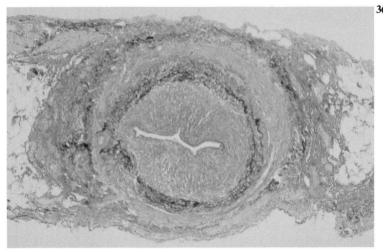

36,37 (a) What histological features are shown in these arterial biopsies from a patient with headache and visual disturbance?
(b) What is the diagnosis? What may be the distribution of the arterial involvement?
(c) What systemic features may be associated, and what treatment is recommended?

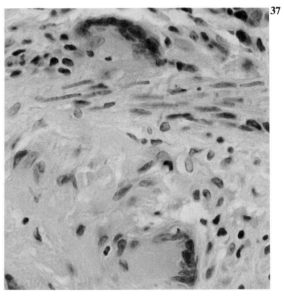

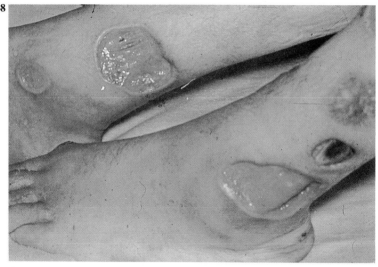

38 A patient presented with rhinorrhoea and nasal ulceration. Chest X-ray revealed patchy parenchymal infiltrate. These ulcerating skin lesions subsequently developed, and were initially necrotic.
(a) What is the diagnosis?
(b) The mean untreated survival in this condition is 5 months—what is the most serious complication?
(c) What form of drug therapy has dramatically improved the prognosis?

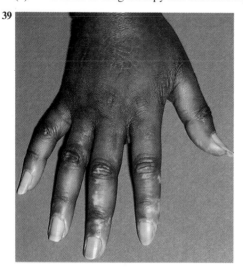

39 A patient complained of progressive stiffness in the fingers with the skin changes demonstrated, and difficulty swallowing.
(a) What is the diagnosis? What three stages are described in the skin change?
(b) What additional skin feature is shown?

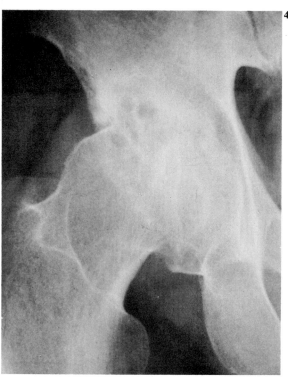

40 Hip X-ray of a 37-year-old man. As well as the arthropathy he had been diagnosed as diabetic 2 years previously, and described loss of body hair and loss of libido. Examination revealed gynaecomastia, testicular atrophy, spider naevi and palmar erythema.

(a) One other skin abnormality was prominent. What was it? What is the diagnosis?

(b) What is believed to be the pathogenesis of this arthropathy? What early radiographic signs may be detected?

(c) What investigations are diagnostic in this condition?

(d) How should this patient be managed?

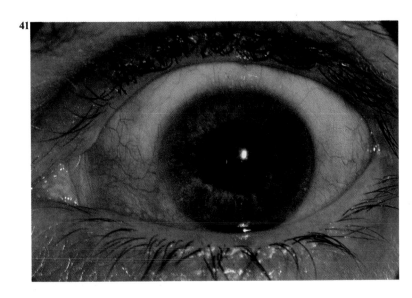

41 This eye sign was observed in a man presenting with inflammatory polyarthritis.
(a) What is the eye involvement?
(b) With what rheumatological condition is this particularly associated?
(c) What is the commonest reason for eye symptoms in rheumatoid arthritis?

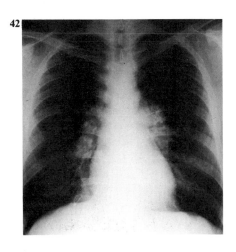

42 A young man presented with an acute arthropathy resulting in warm, red swelling of the ankles.
(a) What diagnosis does this chest X-ray suggest?
(b) What dermatological manifestation of this condition might be anticipated?
(c) What immunological abnormalities are typical of this condition?

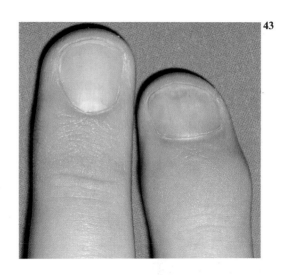

43 (a) What abnormalities are shown in this photograph of the middle and index finger, and what is the diagnosis?
(b) What is the significance of this topographical association?
(c) What factor may trigger activation or osteolytic progression of joint involvement in this condition?

44 A rheumatoid patient complained of difficulty eating and swallowing.
(a) What sign is demonstrated? What is the extra-articular involvement?
(b) What other secretory abnormalities may be symptomatic?
(c) How may a histological diagnosis be simply obtained?

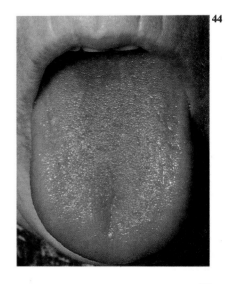

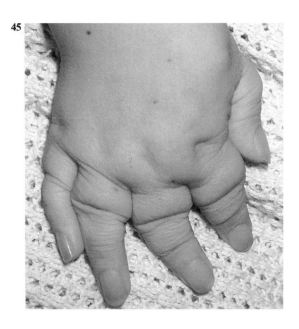

45,46 (a) What is this form of destructive arthropathy?
(b) With what two conditions is it rarely, but typically, associated?
(c) What is the name given to the clinical appearance, and why?

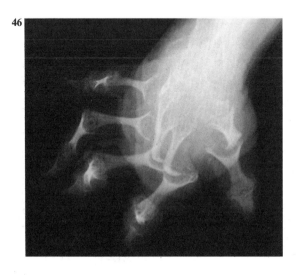

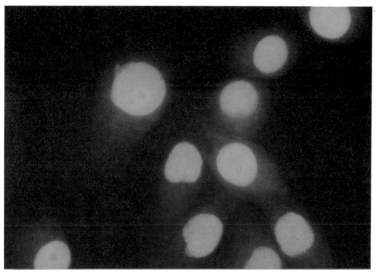

47,48 This indirect immunofluorescence test is performed on a human cell line (or rat liver section) using serum from a patient with a systemic connective tissue disorder.
(a) What is the test?
(b) To what antigenic determinants is this test directed?
(c) What two specific patterns of fluorescence are shown? With what condition is one of these primarily associated?

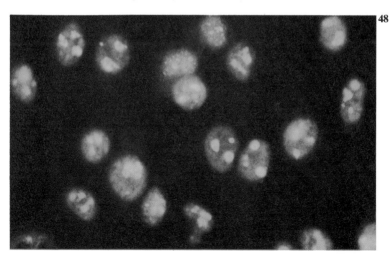

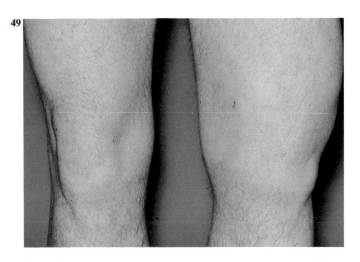

49 Two weeks after an episode of diarrhoea a 19-year-old man rapidly developed this sign in association with pain.
(a) What is this abnormality?
(b) What is the cause? What specific causative agents should be sought?

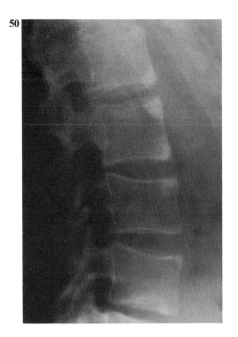

50 (a) What are these radiographic appearances observed in ankylosing spondylitis?
(b) What is the pathological sequence of events resulting in ankylosis of which this lesion forms part?
(c) What other vertebral change may precede syndesmophyte formation?

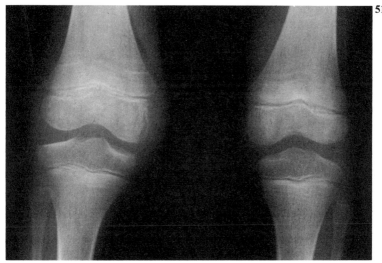

51 A 9-year-old boy had swelling and pain in his right knee and left ankle for 4 years.
(a) Apart from soft tissue swelling, what is the most significant abnormality on the knee X-rays?
(b) What will be the clinical concomitant of these radiographic findings? What treatment may be indicated?
(c) What is the probable diagnosis? What major non-articular complication should be sought?

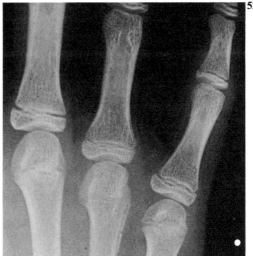

52 What is the most significant abnormality in this hand X-ray of a child with juvenile inflammatory arthritis?

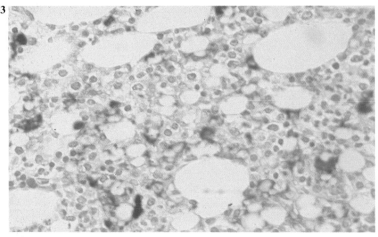

53 A bone marrow biopsy, stained by Perl's reagent, taken from a patient with severe rheumatoid arthritis and haemoglobin 8 g/dl.
(a) What is the most noteworthy observation?
(b) Serum iron was low and serum ferritin very high. What is the explanation for these observations?
(c) What is the most reliable test for iron deficiency in rheumatoid arthritis?

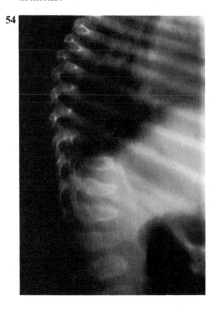

54 A 2½-year-old boy had had active systemic juvenile chronic arthritis for 12 months, which had proved difficult to control.
(a) What abnormality is shown on this spinal X-ray?
(b) What is the most probable cause?
(c) His height was well below the third centile. What is the most important factor in stunting of growth?
(d) If continued corticosteroid therapy is required, how should this be administered?

55 (a) What is this lesion?
(b) For what arthritic condition is it pathognomonic?
(c) What other genitourinary manifestations may this disorder have?

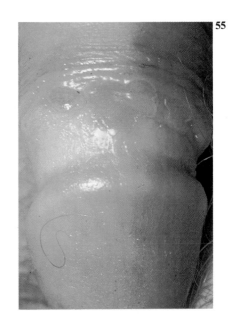

56 A man had an intermittent acute lower limb arthropathy.
(a) What does the photograph show?
(b) Where else would these lesions be expected?
(c) Apart from rheumatoid disease, what other arthropathies may be associated with skin nodule formation?

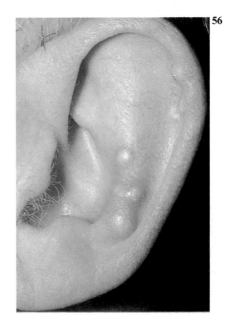

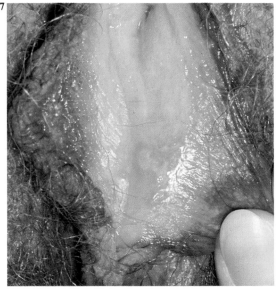

57 A 30-year-old woman presented this lesion in association with intermittent crops of mouth and throat ulcers and large-joint pain.
(a) What abnormality is shown on this photograph of the vulva? What rheumatological diagnosis does this suggest?
(b) What complications of this disorder may be life-threatening?
(c) What investigations may be diagnostically useful?

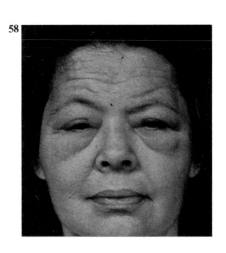

58 A middle-aged woman presented with fever, diffuse rheumatic pain and profound malaise.
(a) What is shown on this clinical photograph?
(b) Her ANF was strongly positive. What two main causes of this appearance should be considered?
(c) What investigations should be requested for diagnosis?

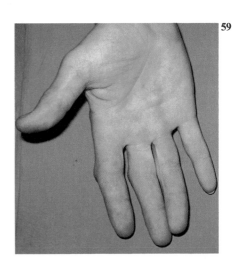

59,60 (a) What two associated abnormalities are shown?
(b) What rheumatological significance do these signs have?

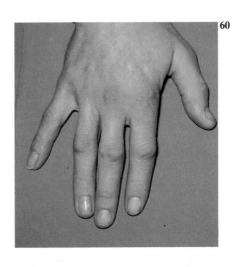

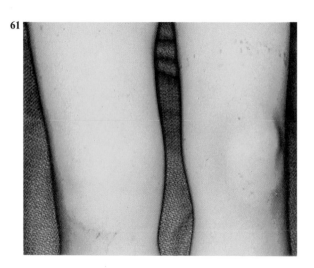

61,62 A 13-year-old girl presented with knee and ankle pain and swelling, and skin rash.
(a) What is the diagnosis?
(b) What is the pathology of the skin rash?
(c) What other organs may be involved? What complications may ensue?
(d) There is seasonal variation in this condition. What predisposing history is often elicited?
(e) How should this patient be managed?

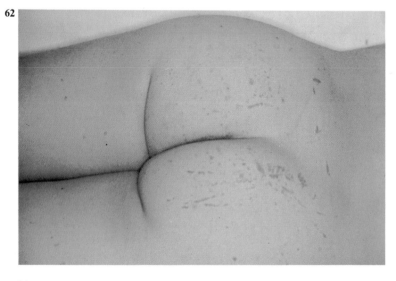

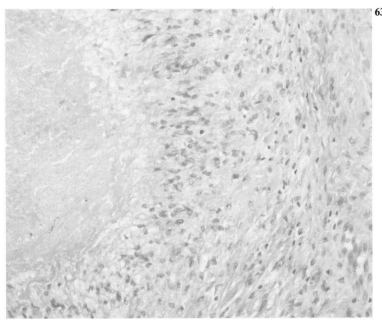

63,64 (a) What histological features are demonstrated in this subcutaneous skin lesion? Of what condition is it diagnostic?
(b) In what other tissues may these lesions be present?
(c) In what other conditions may skin nodules and arthritis be associated?

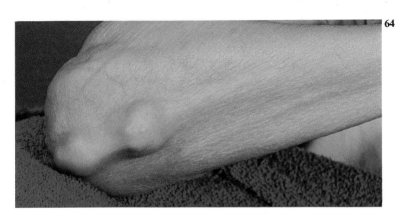

65

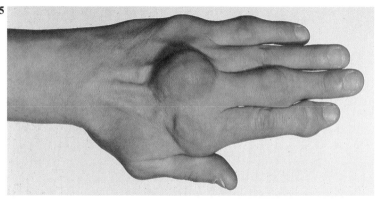

65,66 A man with hand and foot arthropathy and discharging swelling at the elbow was believed to have rheumatoid arthritis.
(a) Which clinical features demonstrated are against this diagnosis?
(b) What is the true diagnosis?
(c) How could this diagnosis be confirmed?
(d) He no longer has acute joint pain and swelling, as he had at presentation. Should any continuous medication be recommended?

66

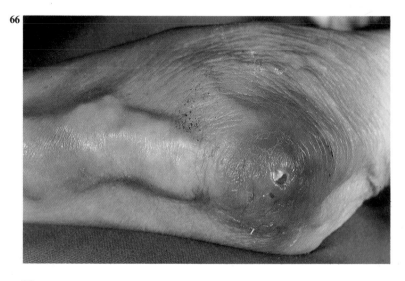

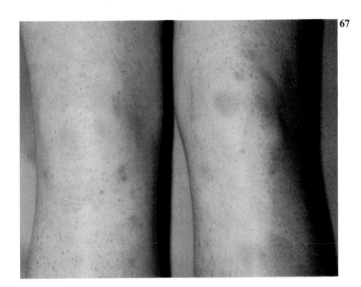

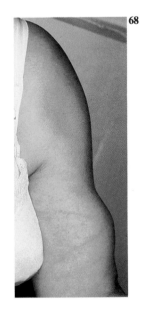

67 A young woman developed very tender red swellings over the lower legs, followed by bilateral knee pain and swelling.
(a) What is the skin disorder?
(b) What medical conditions should be included in the differential diagnosis?
(c) What specific aspects of the history and examination may help to resolve the diagnosis?
(d) What investigations should be requested?

68 A patient complained of acute pain in the arm on lifting a heavy weight, and a swelling developed. What is this traumatically induced condition?

69

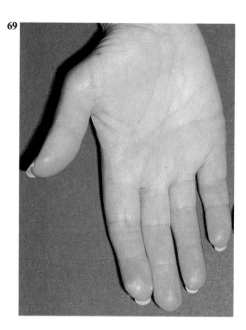

69,70 This photograph and X-ray are from different female patients who both complained of Raynaud's phenomenon commencing as teenagers, and subsequent symptoms included stiffness of the fingers, difficulty in swallowing and some skin markings on the face and hands.

(a) What abnormality is shown?

(b) What other skin abnormalities might be expected?

(c) At what other sites may this abnormality occur?

(d) This collection of symptoms and signs is often associated with a good prognosis. What is this syndrome, and of what disease spectrum does it form part?

70

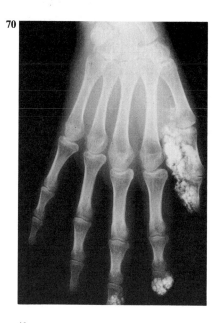

71,72 Joint changes progressing over 15 months.

(a) What is the condition, and what characteristic deformities are shown here?

(b) What other finger deformity is typically associated with the synovitis of these joints?

(c) What surgical procedure may be indicated?

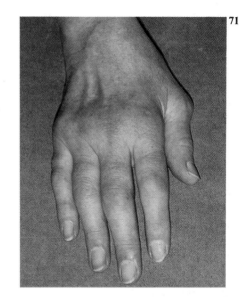

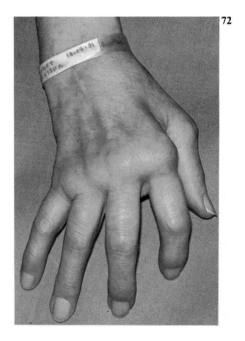

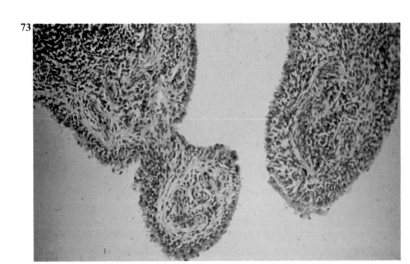

73 (a) What histological features illustrated are characteristic of rheumatoid synovitis?

(b) What immunological cell-types and subtypes might be identified using immunochemical staining?

(c) What cell–cell chemical messengers are believed to be responsible for generating the immunological inflammatory response, and how do they work?

74 A hand X-ray showing early diagnostic evidence of rheumatoid arthritis.

(a) How is the site of the abnormality explained, and what pathological features could be demonstrated at arthrotomy?

(b) What is the place of synovectomy in the management of early rheumatoid arthritis?

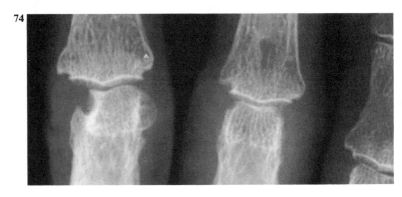

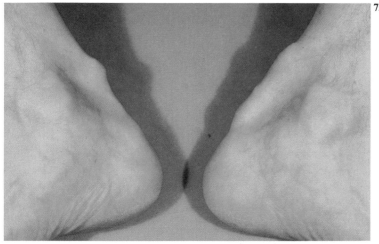

75 (a) What is the probable nature of these firm localised swellings over the heels in a patient with symmetrical inflammatory polyarthritis?
(b) What non-traumatic rheumatological and metabolic conditions may produce inflammatory lesions at this site?

76 The optic fundus of a young woman who presented with acute psychosis. Routine assessment had demonstrated fever, proteinuria and leukopenia.
(a) What retinal abnormalities are shown?
(b) What is the probable diagnosis? What is the pathogenesis of the retinal appearance?
(c) What investigations should be performed to support this diagnosis?

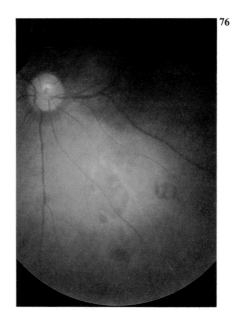

77

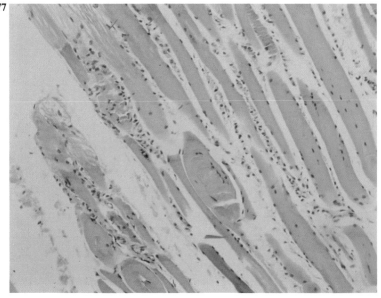

78

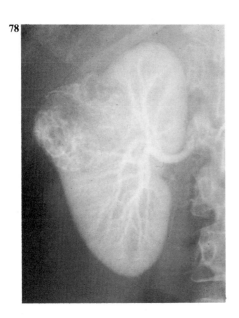

77,78 An histological section and renal angiogram from a patient presenting with muscular weakness, limb pain and fever.

(a) What does the X-ray show?

(b) What does the histological section demonstrate? What is the diagnosis?

(c) How should this patient be managed?

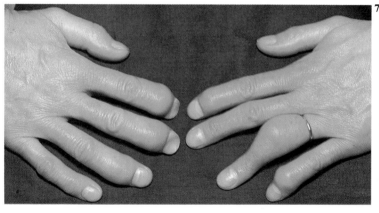

79 A 48-year-old woman's main complaint was of cosmetic hand disfigurement.
(a) What specific arthropathy is suggested by the features shown?
(b) Hand function was well-preserved. What joint-related factors determine loss of hand function in hand arthropathies?

80 A patient receiving penicillamine for rheumatoid arthritis developed these painless skin lesions on minor trauma.
(a) What is the probable cause?
(b) How common is this complication? With what may it be associated?
(c) What is the pathogenesis, and how should it be managed?
(d) How may this complication be prevented?

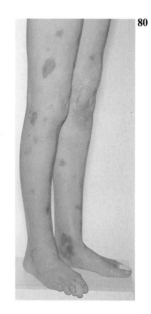

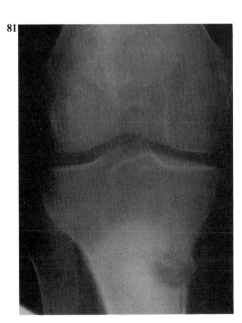

81 (a) What is shown on this X-ray? What is this appearance called?

(b) What is the diagnosis? At what other sites may these bone changes be seen?

(c) What investigations should be requested to support the diagnosis and to elucidate its cause?

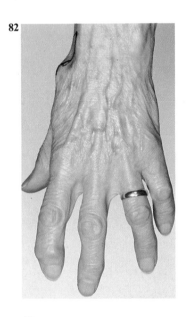

82 (a) What characteristic hand deformity is shown? What other abnormalities are present?

(b) What is the cause of the characteristic deformity? What main functional limitation results?

(c) In which common arthropathy does this deformity typically occur?

83,84 A patient initially presented to an orthopaedic surgeon with recurrent dislocation of the patella and occasional dislocation of the shoulder. Examination also indicated mild scoliosis and pectus carinatum.

(a) What is the significance of the sign demonstrated in **83**?

(b) What helpful diagnostic feature does **84** show?

(c) What is the diagnosis?

(d) What is the probable reason for the thoracic surgical scar?

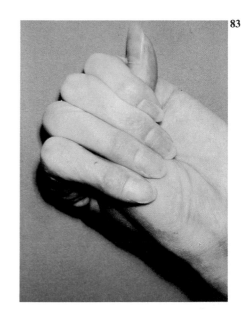

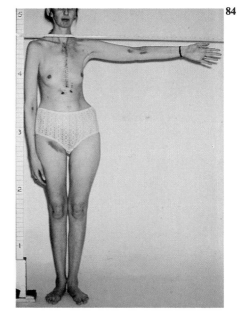

85

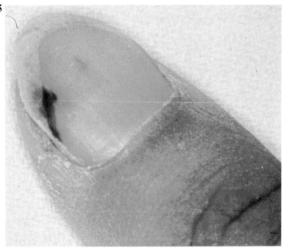

85 (a) What is the nature of this lesion in a patient with rheumatoid arthritis?
(b) What other dermatological manifestations may be a feature of this disease? Where should they be sought?

86

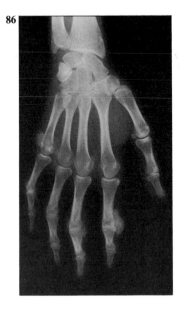

86 An X-ray of the right hand of a patient with chronic renal failure.
(a) What observation can be made?
(b) What biochemical abnormality predisposes most to this condition? What therapies help to counteract it?
(c) At what other non-visceral sites may this occur?
(d) With what clinical rheumatological features may it be associated?

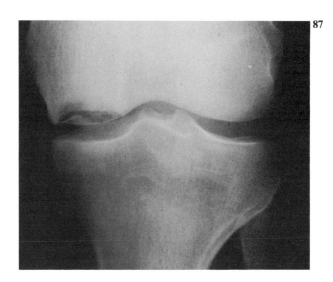

87 A 22-year-old paratrooper complained of progressive discomfort in his knee, markedly aggravated by exercise. He was observed to stand with his knee slightly flexed and foot turned out.
(a) What is the abnormality shown on this X-ray? What is it called?
(b) What is the probable cause? How would this patient best be managed?
(c) At what other sites may this condition occur?

88 A 68-year-old woman presented with fairly acute onset malaise, headache and generalised stiffness.
(a) What can be observed? What would be felt for on palpating this finding?
(b) What specific symptoms should be enquired about?
(c) How should this patient be managed?

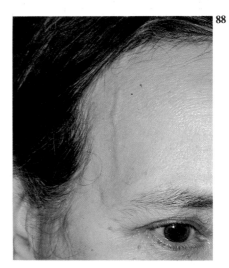

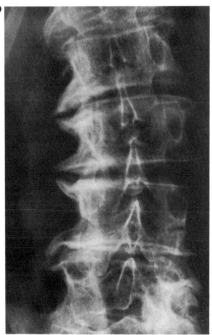

89 (a) What main bony changes can be observed on this lumbar spine X-ray?
(b) What is the condition?
(c) What differentiates syndesmophytes from vertebral osteophytes?

90 A 43-year-old hypertensive man had developed acute pain at the base of the great toe 2 weeks previously.
(a) What signs can be observed?
(b) What is the diagnosis?
(c) He had one previous attack 18 months earlier. What drug treatment should be recommended?

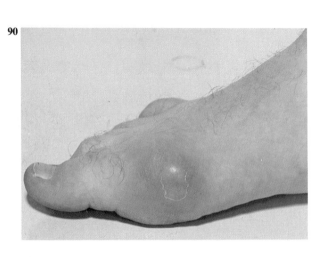

91 (a) What three diagnostic features are shown in this X-ray of a man with spinal stiffness?
(b) What is the diagnosis?

92 X-rays taken 3 weeks after the onset of acute painful swelling of the left wrist with rigors and fever.
(a) What is the diagnosis?
(b) What is the most likely causative agent?
(c) What initial treatment regime should be offered?
(d) What additional measure might have prevented this degree of cartilage loss?

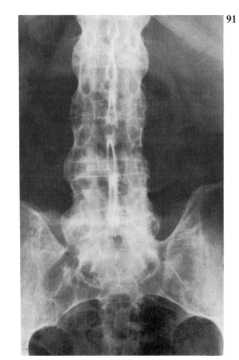

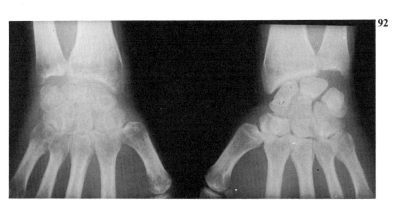

93

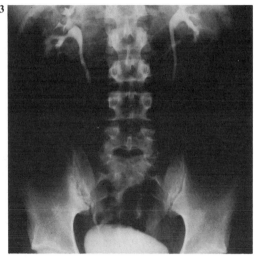

93 A young man presented with asymptomatic microscopic haematuria at a routine employment medical.
(a) What abnormality is shown on this X-ray?
(b) What explanations should be considered for the haematuria in view of these X-ray appearances?

94

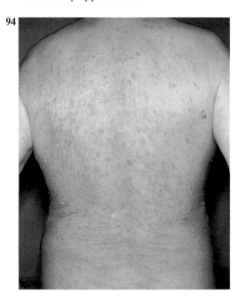

94 A scaly pruritic skin rash developed in a rheumatoid patient receiving second-line therapy.
(a) What is the probable cause? Is this appearance typical?
(b) This man had responded well to second-line therapy. How should the patient now be managed?

95,96 An elderly woman complained of back pain and weight loss in addition to arm pain. Investigations demonstrated anaemia and hypercalcaemia. The smear shows her bone marrow aspirate.

(a) What is the probable diagnosis? Apart from the back, what other area should be X-rayed?

(b) What does the bone marrow smear show?

(c) An arthropathy resulting from synovial infiltration is sometimes associated with this condition. What is the nature of this complication?

(d) What criteria determine the need for specific treatment in this condition?

(e) What precaution must be exercised in investigating patients with this condition?

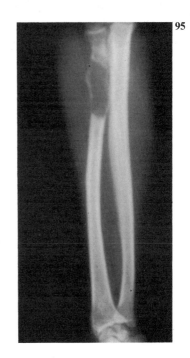

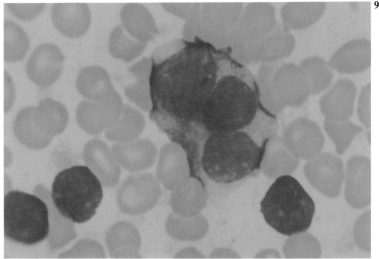

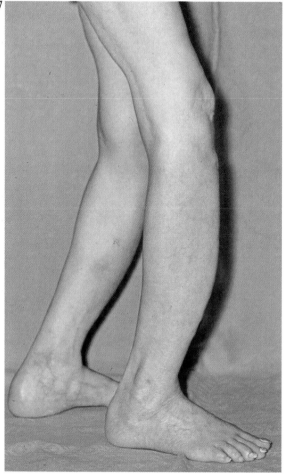

97,98 (a) What is the cause of this deformity?
(b) What drugs are specific for this condition?
(c) What laboratory measures could be used to monitor
response to treatment?
(d) Is hypercalcaemia a feature of this condition?

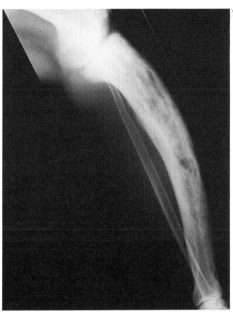

99 A young man developed persistent bilateral heel pain on walking, following an acute inflammatory arthropathy involving a knee, both ankles and the right third toe. He complained of eye soreness at initial presentation.
(a) What abnormality is shown on this X-ray?
(b) What is the probable diagnosis? What form of eye involvement occurs in this condition?

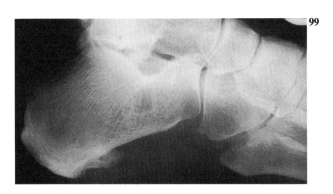

100

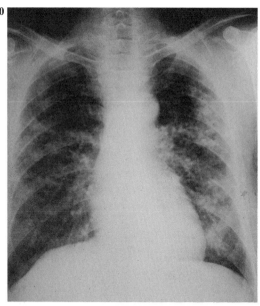

100,101 Chest X-rays taken 2 years apart on a miner with rheumatoid arthritis who had to take early retirement due to progressive breathlessness.

(a) What features can be seen on the earlier X-ray, and what subsequent changes have taken place?

101

(b) What is the relationship between his job and his initial X-ray?

(c) What eponym is given to the lung abnormality resulting from this association?

102, 103 (a) What skin abnormalities do these two patients with rheumatoid arthritis have?

(b) What complication do these signs represent? What serological abnormalities may be associated with its occurrence?

(c) What other extra-articular manifestations of rheumatoid disease may be due to this pathological process?

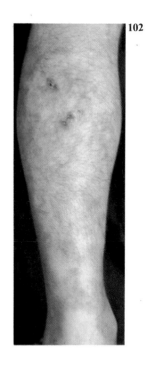

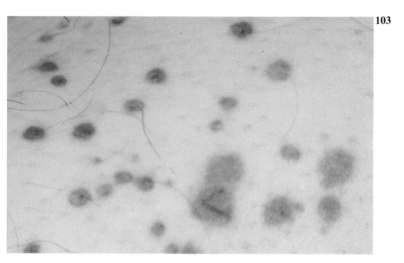

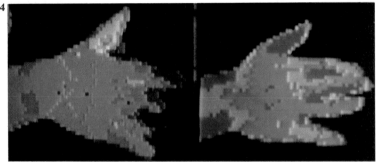

104 A patient with polymyositis has been asked to immerse one hand in ice-cold water.
(a) What investigation is illustrated? What abnormality is demonstrated?
(b) For what other aspect of rheumatological investigation has this procedure been recommended? What are its main drawbacks?

105 (a) What diagnosis does the clinical appearance of this hand suggest?
(b) What pathological process causes the skin changes over the third PIP joint and wrist? In what other ways may this process manifest?
(c) What cardiac complications may occur?

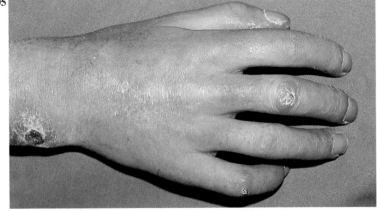

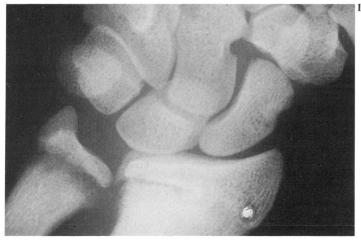

106 An Asian girl presented with tender, bony swelling at wrists and ankles.
(a) What diagnosis does this X-ray suggest?
(b) What laboratory parameters would be helpful in supporting this diagnosis?
(c) What would be the simplest way of confirming the diagnosis?

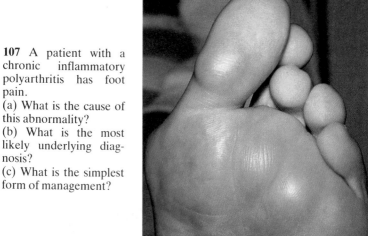

107 A patient with a chronic inflammatory polyarthritis has foot pain.
(a) What is the cause of this abnormality?
(b) What is the most likely underlying diagnosis?
(c) What is the simplest form of management?

108

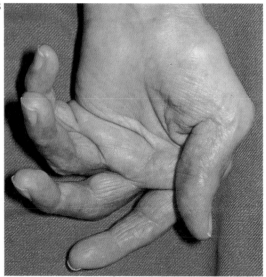

108 A patient with rheumatoid arthritis has brown skin pigmentation, particularly marked over the anterior shins.
(a) With what extra-articular manifestations is this sign particularly associated?
(b) An additional feature in this patient was repeated severe infection. What treatments should be considered for this complication?
(c) With what other skin manifestation is this condition associated?

109 A child started to limp with thigh pain.
(a) What is the diagnosis?
(b) What is the aetiology and pathogenesis of this condition?
(c) What is the typical age and sex of this disorder?
(d) What management should be recommended?

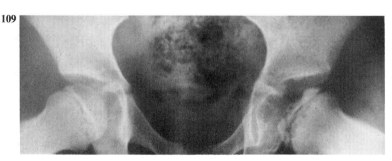

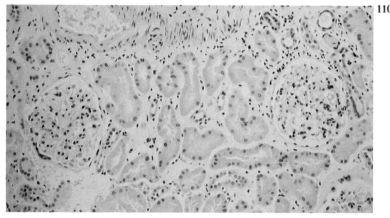

110 A 13-year-old boy with a 7-year history of persistent systemic onset juvenile arthritis developed ankle swelling. Heavy proteinuria was noted.
(a) What clinical complication has occurred, and what specific cause does the renal biopsy indicate?
(b) What specific drug treatment should be considered for this complication? What serious long-term side-effects may result from this treatment?
(c) What other biopsy sites may confirm this diagnosis?

111 (a) What abnormality is shown in this knee X-ray of an elderly patient? What is its precise location?
(b) The patient presented with painful swelling of the MCP and PIP joints symmetrically. What is the probable relationship between the radiographic abnormality in the knee and these symptoms?

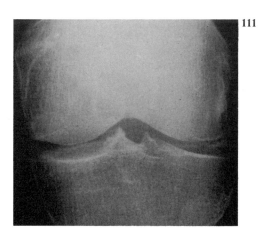

112 A 47-year-old man with degenerative arthropathy of the cervical spine (cervical spondylosis).
(a) What abnormality is shown on this oblique radiograph?
(b) What is the precise pathogenesis of this specific abnormality?
(c) What would dictate the management of this patient?

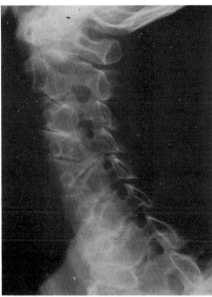

113 (a) What is the cause of the abnormal appearances of these ischial bones?
(b) What other major radiological abnormalities are demonstrated? What is the diagnosis?

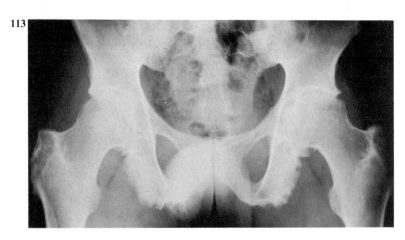

114 A patient with osteoarthrosis had been particularly troubled by hand pain and had developed some functional difficulty.

(a) What is the most striking abnormality shown?

(b) What is the most likely cause of this?

(c) What other general medical conditions should be considered in this patient?

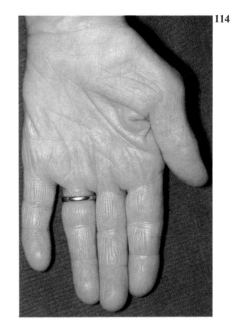

115 A young man initially presented with acute swelling of the left knee following trauma at the age of 18 months. The knee was warm and extremely painful, and he was febrile. Subsequent joint involvement had been acute, short-lived swelling recurring in the same knee, the elbow and ankle.

(a) What diagnoses should be considered at the initial presentation at 18 months?

(b) What specific questions should be asked at the initial presentation?

(c) At presentation the diagnosis was suggested by a strong family history affecting males only, and subsequent episodes have been partially aborted by specific replacement therapy. What is the diagnosis?

(d) What are the major signs demonstrated in this radiograph?

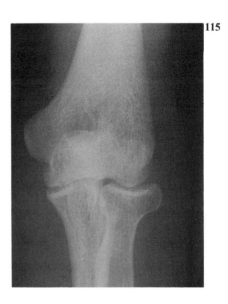

116

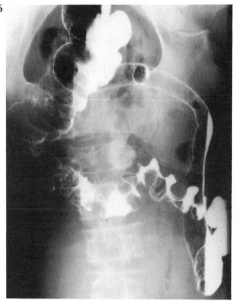

A 37-year-old woman became ill with painful swelling of both knees, left ankle and left wrist, mouth ulceration, tender skin swellings over the shins and increased stool frequency. She gave a past history of intermittent increased stool frequency.

(a) What does this barium enema show?

(b) Is a temporal relationship between joint involvement and this gastro-intestinal abnormality typical?

(c) What skin abnormality has been described? What other systemic abnormalities may complicate this condition?

(d) What aetiological theories may explain these associations?

117

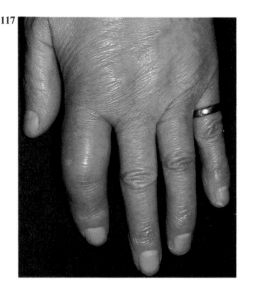

117 (a) What is the main clinical feature shown?

(b) What is the term given to this type of involvement from inflammatory arthropathy, and with what conditions is it particularly associated?

(c) Name three structures which may be involved by the inflammatory process. What unusual radiographic feature may be present?

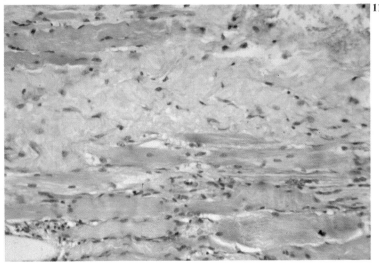

118 A muscle biopsy taken from a patient with muscle wasting and weakness following a 2-year history of severe polymyositis.
(a) What significant abnormalities are shown?
(b) How should this information guide further treatment?

119 A 67-year-old woman rapidly developed a painful, swollen and red shoulder over 24 h, and was found to have a temperature of 37.5°C.
(a) What two diagnoses should you consider?
(b) Her blood white cell count was normal. What two diagnostic investigations should be performed?
(c) Radiography showed linear opacity outlining the hyaline cartilage of the humeral head. What substance causes this appearance?
(d) What would be expected in the synovial fluid?
(e) Which joint is most commonly affected by this condition? At which three sites is the radiographic feature most commonly seen?

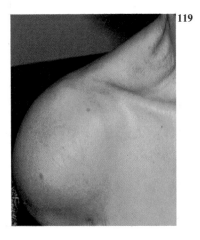
119

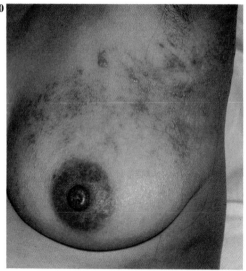

120 A patient with systemic lupus erythematosus developed severe pain under the arm followed by this vesicular haemorrhagic rash.
(a) What is the cause of the rash?
(b) How can the diagnosis be urgently confirmed?
(c) The previously-established treatment included corticosteroids and azathioprine. How should the rash be treated?

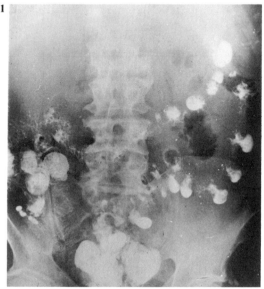

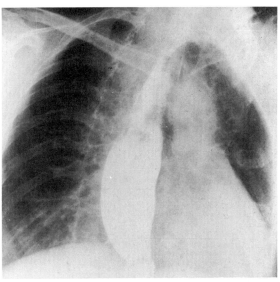

121, 122 Two barium contrast studies showing two of the gastro-intestinal abnormalities of a systemic connective tissue disease.

(a) What abnormality is demonstrated in **122**? What two symptoms may result?

(b) What abnormality is demonstrated in **121**? What potential complications may result?

(c) What is the diagnosis?

(d) What is commonest manifestation of small bowel involvement in this condition?

123

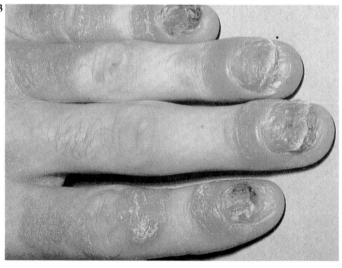

123 These dermatological changes developed over 3 weeks in association with more-extensive changes on the feet, disabling pain in the right 1st metatarso phalangeal joint and hind foot, and urethral discharge. What is the diagnosis? What is this skin abnormality?

124 A skin rash over the trunk observed in a young child admitted with swinging fever and swelling of the hands, wrists and knees.

(a) What is the most likely diagnosis? What other diagnoses should be considered?

(b) A persistent inflammatory polyarthritis developed, associated with fever. What other clinical signs of systemic disease may be observed in this condition?

(c) Systemic corticosteroids have been used for this condition. What side effects may result? How can these be reduced?

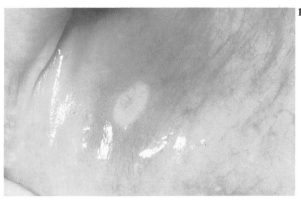

125 This mouth lesion was demonstrated during follow-up of treatment for rheumatoid arthritis.
(a) With what two second-line drugs is this associated?
(b) What other routine monitoring must be performed during administration of these drugs?

126 A young woman presented with acute knee and ankle pain, eye discomfort and tender red swellings on the shins.
(a) What is the most likely diagnosis?
(b) At what site in the eye is the inflammation in this patient? What is the more characteristic ocular involvement in this condition?
(c) In the absence of eye involvement, what other cause for the presenting signs and symptoms should be considered?
(d) What related clinical and radiographic signs may help to differentiate?

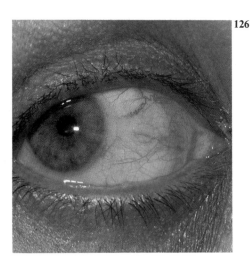

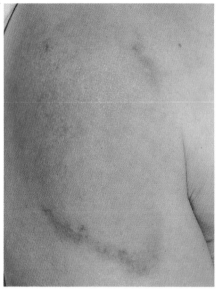

127 A 35-year-old woman with an 18-month history of painful swelling in the right shoulder, believed to be post-traumatic after an earlier aspiration demonstrated dark brown fluid suggesting old blood. There is no other evidence of a bleeding disorder.

(a) This clinical appearance developed spontaneously. What diagnosis does it suggest?

(b) Arthroscopy yielded the diagnosis which was confirmed by histology. What were the arthroscopic appearances?

(c) The shoulder is an unusual site for this condition. What is the commonest presentation?

(d) What is the treatment?

128 Material discharging from what was believed to be an infected skin lesion on the foot, viewed under polarised-light microscopy.

(a) What can be observed?

(b) What is the significance of this sign? How is this fact used diagnostically?

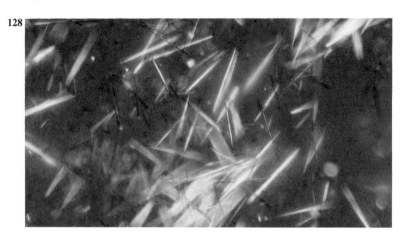

129 A young man presented with fever, a sore mouth and pain in his hands, feet and ankles.
(a) What abnormalities are shown?
(b) What is the diagnosis? How could this be confirmed?
(c) What other causes of articular pain should be considered in this group of conditions?

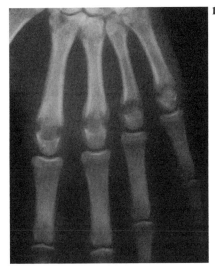

130 Following myocardial infarction treated at home a 68-year-old man developed swelling and burning pain in the left hand, with pain and limitation of shoulder movement.
(a) What abnormalities are shown? What is the name of this syndrome?
(b) What other skin signs and symptoms may be present?
(c) What radiographic features would be expected in this case?
(d) Name three other medical conditions which may give rise to this syndrome?

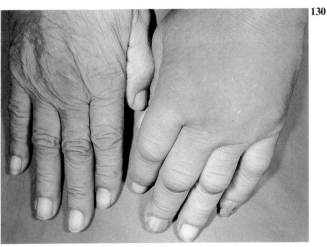

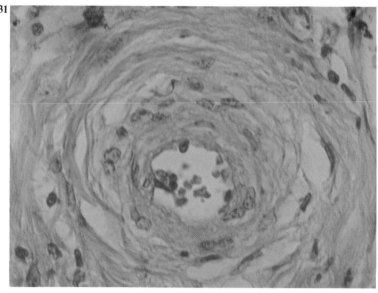

131 This histological appearance was observed in a spleen surgically removed from a patient presenting with fever, lymphadenopathy and pancytopenia.
(a) What can be observed, and what is the probable diagnosis?
(b) What is the aetiology of this appearance?

132

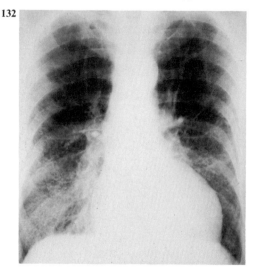

132 A middle-aged man presented with breathlessness on exertion and arthralgia. Positive rheumatoid factor was demonstrated.
(a) What pathological process does the radiograph suggest? What diagnoses should be considered?
(b) What forms of therapy should be considered?

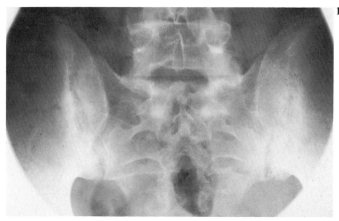

133 A 28-year-old bus driver had an 18-month history of low back pain and stiffness which initially followed a 10-day bout of bloody diarrhoea. He also had pain in the soles of both feet on walking, and episodic conjunctivitis.
(a) What abnormalities are demonstrated in this X-ray?
(b) What is the most likely diagnosis? What differential diagnoses should be considered?
(c) What is the probable explanation for the foot pain? What local treatment may be beneficial?

134 This facial appearance developed while on holiday, in a young woman whose only previous symptom had been mild intermittent arthralgia and hair loss.
(a) What is the diagnosis?
(b) What investigations should be performed for diagnosis and assessment?
(c) What advice should be given for future holidays?

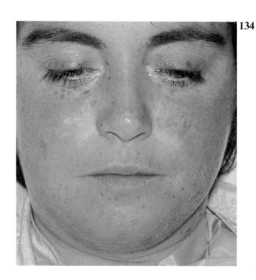

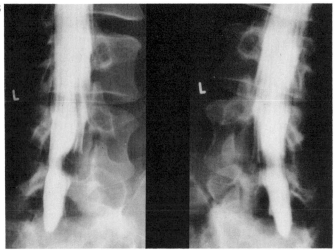

135 X-ray showing the 4th and 5th lumbar vertebrae of a young labourer presenting with sciatic pain following a back injury while lifting.
(a) What abnormality does the myelogram show?
(b) How should this patient be managed initially?
(c) What are the indications for surgical intervention for this condition?

136 (a) What is the most likely cause of these skin lesions in a 65-year-old woman receiving drug treatment for rheumatoid arthritis?
(b) What is the probable pathogenesis? In what other tissue may this be a problem?

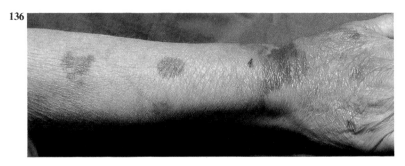

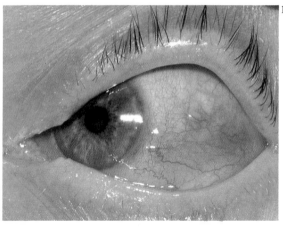

137 A patient with rheumatoid arthritis.
(a) What abnormalities can be observed in the eye?
(b) What serious complication may result?

138 (a) What is the bilateral pelvic deformity shown in this X-ray?
(b) What is the commonest cause of this deformity? Name two other conditions which may cause it?
(c) How may this X-ray influence decisions about further management?

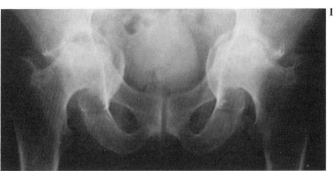

138

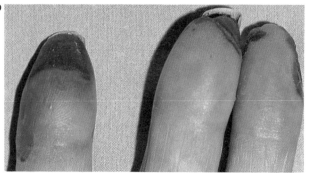

139 (a) What is the cause of this uncommon complication of rheumatoid disease?
(b) What treatments have been recommended?

140 A painful inflammatory eye condition followed the development of an inflammatory monoarthritis in a 33-year-old man.
(a) What signs are shown?
(b) What is the eye condition?
(c) With what group of arthropathies is this condition associated? What single radiographic investigation may help in diagnosis?

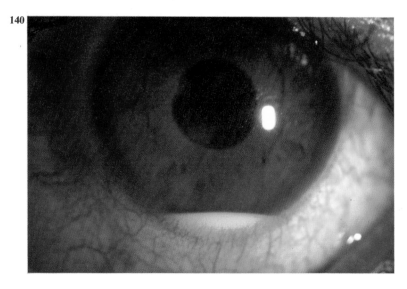

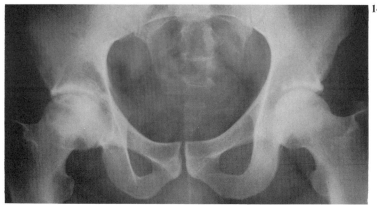

141 A 35-year-old man presented with right groin pain and a limp.
(a) What abnormalities are shown? What is the nature of this abnormality?
(b) Name three predisposing factors? What biochemical test should be performed?
(c) What is the prognosis for this patient?

142 A 70-year-old man complained of back pain.
(a) What observation can be made?
(b) What two main diagnoses should be considered?
(c) What laboratory test may help to differentiate these two?
(d) Would a bone scan be useful?

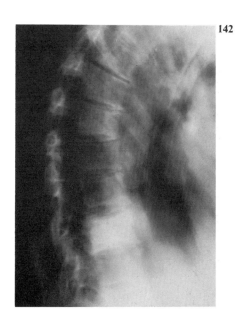

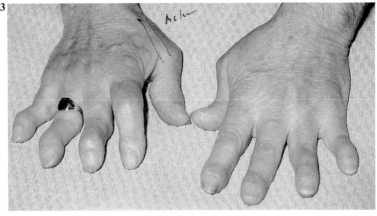

143 (a) What deformities are shown in these hands of a patient with psoriatic arthritis?
(b) What joint involvement suggests that the arthritis is not rheumatoid?

144 (a) What does this arthrogram on a patient with early rheumatoid arthritis show?
(b) In what other conditions may arthrography be useful?

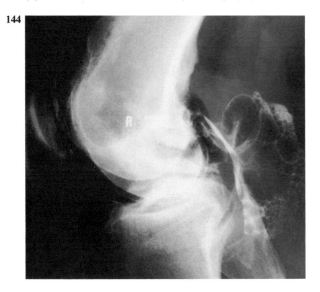

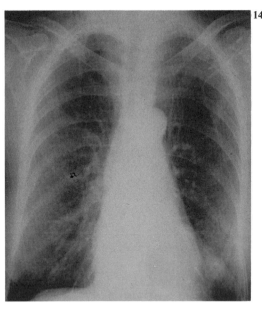

145 A chest X-ray performed routinely on a 60-year-old woman with active rheumatoid disease.
(a) What abnormality is shown?
(b) What diagnoses should be considered?
(c) How should the patient be investigated?

146 A young man had juvenile onset arthritis as a young child.
(a) What complication has resulted?
(b) With what other skeletal involvement may this be associated?
(c) What difficulty may this pose during later medical care?

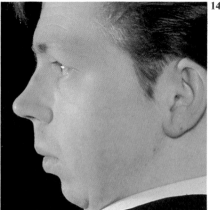

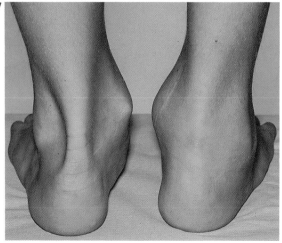

147,148 A young merchant seaman with a previous ankle injury presented with heel pain of 10 weeks' duration.
(a) What abnormality is shown in **147**?
(b) What relevant abnormality does **148** show?
(c) What diagnoses should be considered? What specific symptoms should be enquired about?
(d) What specific treatment should be considered?

148

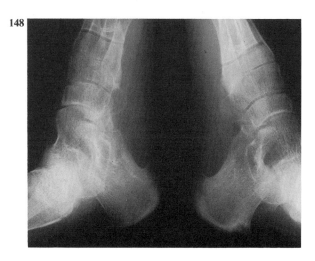

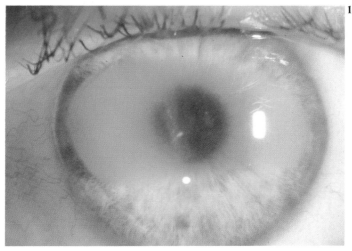

149 (a) What can be seen in this eye? What is this condition called?
(b) With what type of arthropathy is this complication associated?
(c) What steps could be taken to prevent this occurrence?

150 A middle-aged woman described changes in the skin of her distal arms and legs, and breathlessness on exertion.

(a) What abnormalities are shown?

(b) What is the probable cause?

(c) What is the most sensitive measure of the associated lung abnormality? What respiratory investigations should be monitored during follow-up of this patient?

(d) What therapies have been shown to arrest the lung damage in this condition?

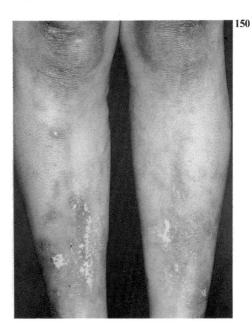

151

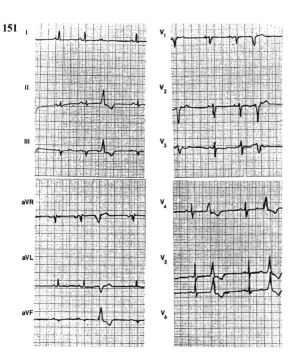

151 An ECG performed on a patient with rheumatoid arthritis who complained of tiredness, breathlessness and ankle oedema.

(a) What is the most significant abnormality and the probable cause?

(b) What clinical signs will help to support this diagnosis?

(c) What other unrelated disorder may give this ECG appearance?

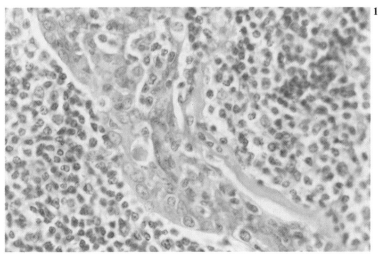

152 A swollen parotid salivary gland excised for diagnosis.
(a) What is the most prominent cell type in this section? What additional histological feature is shown?
(b) Further questioning elicited a history of symmetrical hand and feet joint pain and swelling. What is the probable cause of the parotid swelling? What other symptoms are commonly present?
(c) What other organs may be involved by the exocrine function abnormalities in this condition?
(d) What late life-threatening complication may result from this condition?

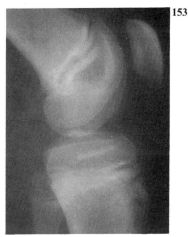

153 A teenage boy presented with knee pain during exercise. No evidence of synovitis could be demonstrated.
(a) What abnormality is shown on this X-ray? What is the eponym given to this condition?
(b) At what age does this condition occur? What predisposing factors have been implicated?

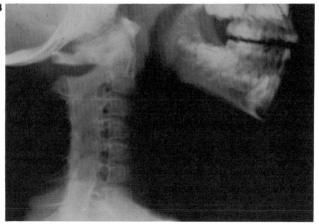

154 A young adult had recovered from an inflammatory polyarthropathy commencing at the age of 5 years.
What abnormality does this X-ray show?

155,156 A young man with spinal pain and stiffness.
(a) What is the probable diagnosis?
(b) What abnormalities are shown on the cervical spine X-ray?
(c) What do these changes represent? What other patterns of arthropathy are associated with this skin condition?

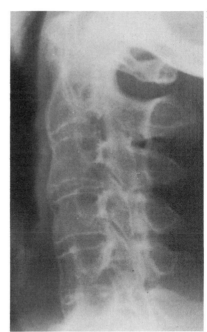

157 A patient with scleroderma.
(a) What two abnormalities are shown in this radiograph?
(b) At what other sites may bone changes be observed?

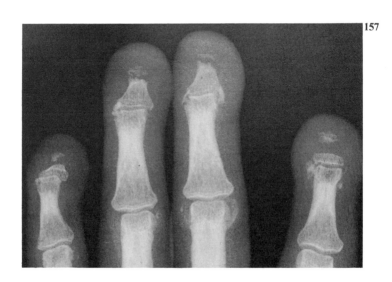

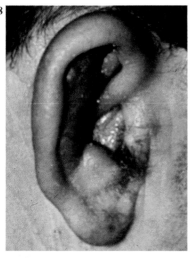

158,159 A 45-year-old man initially presented 9 months previously with this swollen, red and extremely tender ear pinna. Collapse of the nasal bridge (similar to that shown) developed painlessly and gradually about 4 months later.

(a) What is the diagnosis?

(b) The patient has developed vertigo. What is the cause of this?

(c) What other sensory organ may be affected?

(d) What two potentially fatal complications may occur in this disorder?

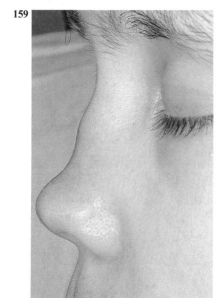

160,161 (a) What abnormalities are shown on these X-rays representing early and late stages of an interphalangeal arthropathy? (b) With what condition is this type of arthropathy typically associated?

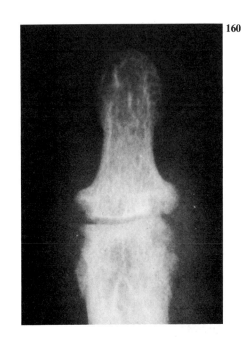

160

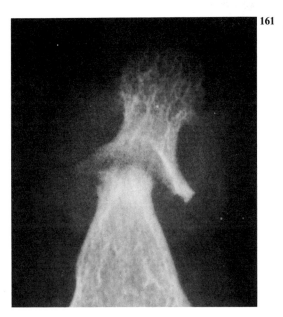

161

162

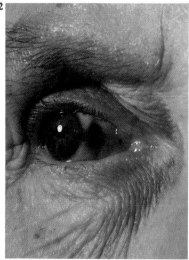

162–164 A patient developed early large-joint degenerative arthropathy with spinal limitation at an early age.
(a) What is the most striking abnormality of the intervertebral joint?
(b) What sign is shown in the eye?
(c) What is the connection between these three photographs?
(d) What is the inheritance of this disorder?

163

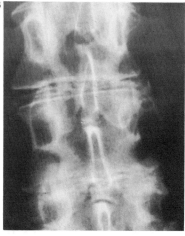

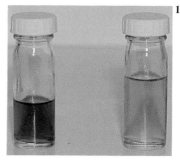

165 An elderly patient presented with deteriorating vision and confusion and generalised aching, and a markedly elevated ESR was obtained on blood testing.

(a) What two diagnoses are suggested by the presenting features? Which does this skull X-ray confirm?

(b) How could the diagnosis be confirmed?

(c) What was the cause of the deteriorating vision and confusion, and how should it be treated?

(d) What specific therapy should be given for this condition?

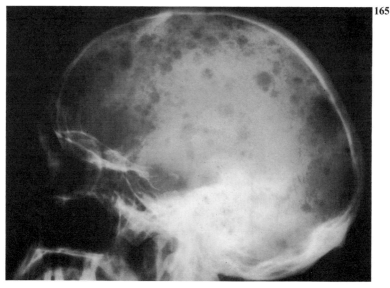

166

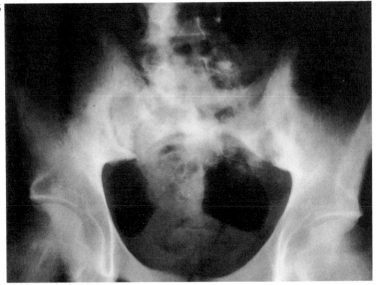

166 A middle-aged man had a 5-month history of progressive pain in the left low back and groin. He felt generally unwell and had lost weight.
(a) What is shown on the X-ray?
(b) What is the probable diagnosis?
(c) Detail the drug regime needed?

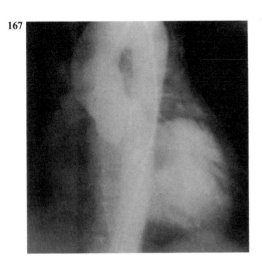

167 (a) What is the significance of this appearance following injection of contrast into the aorta in a patient with rheumatoid disease?
(b) What is the pathology of this complication in rheumatoid disease? How does it differ from that found in ankylosing spondylitis?
(c) What other cardiac complications may occur in rheumatoid disease?

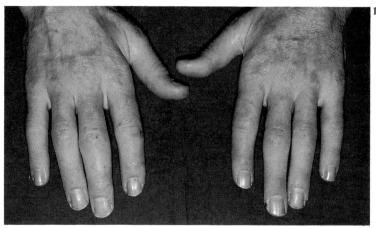

168 A 64-year-old man developed progressive aching, particularly in the limb girdles, and weakness most marked on descending stairs and standing from a low chair.
(a) What signs can be observed in his hands?
(b) What is the probable diagnosis, and what investigations should be performed?
(c) What disease associations may this condition have in the adult population?

169 A young teenager presented with acutely painful swelling of several large joints in a migratory pattern.
(a) What is the dermatological abnormality? What is the probable diagnosis?
(b) What investigations would support this diagnosis?
(c) What major neurological complication may rarely occur?

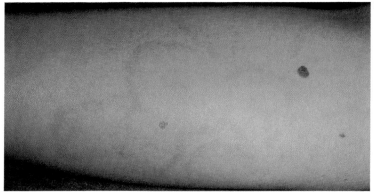

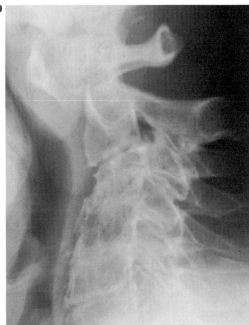

170 (a) What is the major abnormality on this cervical spine X-ray?
(b) What complications may result?

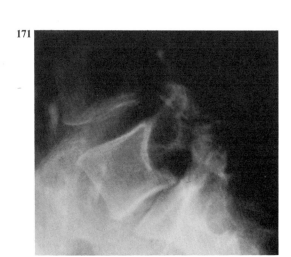

171,172 A patient with a long history of pain in the calf and foot.

(a) What vertebral abnormality is shown?

(b) What clinical signs shown indicate the cause?

(c) What other spinal abnormality may be present in this condition?

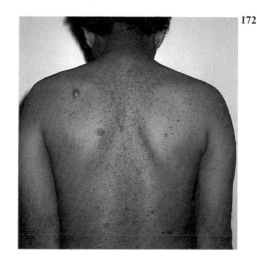

173 A 33-year-old man with a history of previous calf vein thrombosis and pustular, acne-like skin lesions attended with several painful mouth ulcers, clouding of vision and joint pain in the wrists, knees and ankles.

(a) What is the diagnosis? What other dermatological manifestations should be asked about or sought?

(b) What is the significance of the venous thrombosis history?

(c) What specific ophthalmic sign visible to the naked eye should be sought? What ophthalmic pathology may result in visual loss?

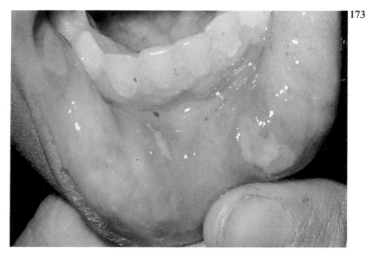

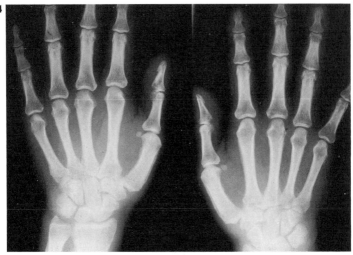

174 A man had been treated with radioactive iodine for Grave's disease 5 years previously. He developed pain in the hands and feet with soft tissue swelling.
(a) What abnormality does the hand X-ray show?
(b) What is this condition? With what other clinical signs may it be associated?
(c) With what abnormal laboratory feature of Grave's disease is this condition typically associated?

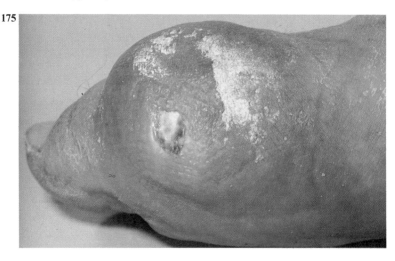

175,176 An elderly woman, provisionally diagnosed as having osteoarthrosis, was referred for treatment of presumed infected bunion.
(a) What can be seen in **175**?
(b) What is the diagnosis? What clue is present in **176**?
(c) What drug treatment is commonly responsible for precipitating this condition in the elderly?

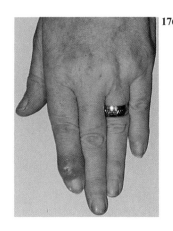

177 A 33-year-old man presented with a 10-week history of symmetrical inflammatory-type joint symptoms and breathlessness on exertion.
(a) What radiographic features are shown in the chest X-ray?
(b) Is this a feature of rheumatoid arthritis?
(c) The diagnosis in this patient was confirmed on histological examination of liver biopsy. What were the findings?
(d) Name two blood investigations which may help to differentiate this condition from rheumatoid arthritis?

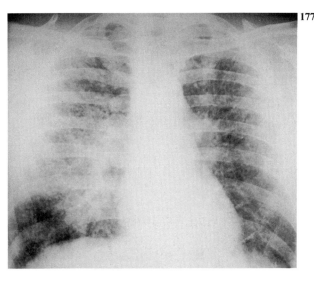

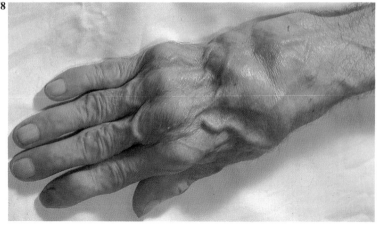

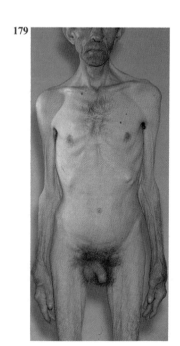

178,179 A man with severe rheumatoid arthritis complained of intermittent fever, weight loss and increased swelling of wrist, knee and ankle.

(a) What complication should first be considered as the cause of these additional symptoms?

(b) Name three factors predisposing patients with rheumatoid arthritis to this complication?

(c) What signs or investigations normally associated with this condition may be absent or normal in rheumatoid patients?

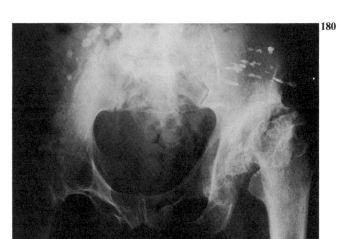

180 An elderly woman previously had a septic arthritis of the right hip, and had become progressively disabled due to painless limitation of left hip movement.
(a) What has been the result of the right hip septic arthritis?
(b) What abnormal features are demonstrated in the left hip joint? What is the probable cause, and what important clue is also evident?

181 (a) What are the skin lesions over this patient's knee?
(b) The patient's first rheumatic symptom was an acute migratory arthropathy as a young teenager, resembling rheumatic fever. What is the precise diagnosis?
(c) What is the untreated life-expectancy in this condition?
(d) What advice would you give this patient's family?

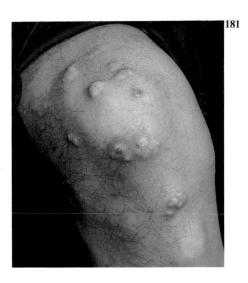

182

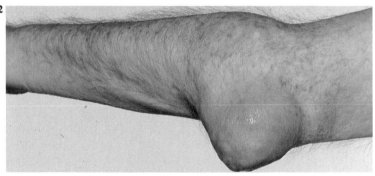

182 (a) What abnormality of the elbow is shown?
(b) This patient has rheumatoid arthritis. What additional abnormality may be associated with this swelling?
(c) What treatment should be recommended?

183

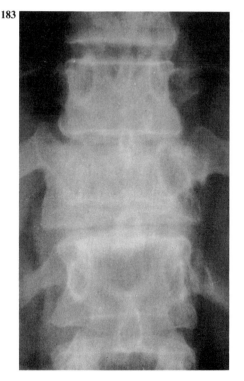

183,184 A 52-year-old woman presented with insidious-onset back and hip pain of duration 2 years.
(a) What abnormalities are demonstrated on the bone scan and X-ray?
(b) What is the most likely diagnosis? What alternatives should be considered?
(c) What investigations should be performed in this case?

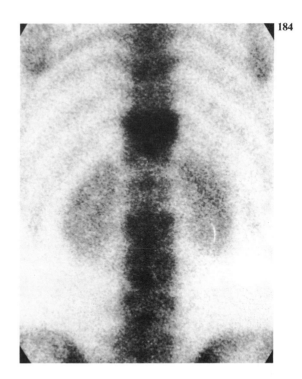

184

185 A patient presented with fever, malaise and abdominal pain, and progressed to develop bilateral foot drop and paraesthesia in the ulna border of the left forearm.

(a) What does this slide show?

(b) What is the diagnosis in this patient?

(c) What determines the prognosis in this condition?

(d) What treatment should be recommended?

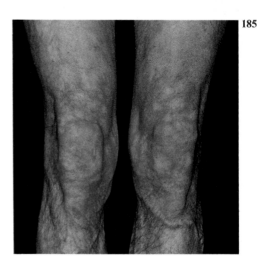

185

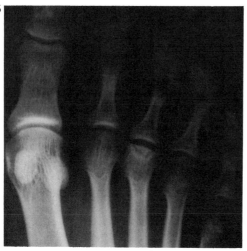

186 An 18-year-old man complained of pain, tenderness and swelling in the region of the third metatarso-phalangeal joint.

(a) What abnormality can be seen on the X-ray? What is the probable pathogenic process responsible?

(b) What eponym is given to this condition?

(c) What late complications may follow?

187 An 11-year-old boy presented with pain and swelling of wrists, knees and ankles, with fever, malaise and this rash.

(a) What is the probable diagnosis?

(b) What additional clinical signs are useful in diagnosing this condition particularly in childhood?

(c) How could the diagnosis be confirmed?

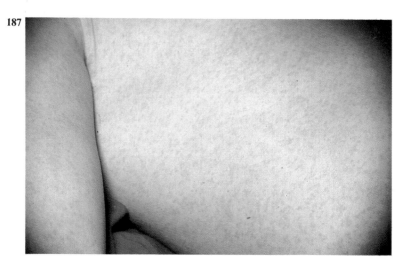

188 A young woman became stunted during childhood due to bone damage, and became deaf during her early teens.
(a) What is the diagnosis?
(b) What additional clinical features may aid diagnosis?
(c) This heterogenous condition is genetically determined. What is the pathogenetic defect?

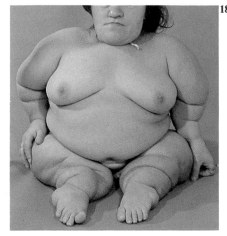

189 A middle-aged Jamaican man had relatively pain-free finger deformity-associated purple nodular skin lesions.
(a) What is the diagnosis?
(b) What are the skin lesions called?
(c) Apart from an acute arthropathy, with what other musculoskeletal involvement may this condition present?

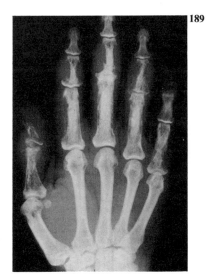

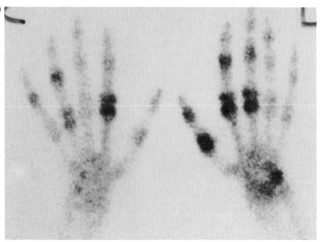

190 A technetium–99m phosphonate scan of the hands of a young woman with arthralgia of uncertain cause.
(a) What abnormality is shown?
(b) To what are the abnormalities due? What is the probable diagnosis?
(c) What other conditions may cause a 'hot' scan?

191,192 A 42-year-old woman with a long history of moderate arthralgia.
(a) What can be seen in the clinical photograph of the hand?
(b) What radiographic abnormality can be seen?
(c) What is the most likely diagnosis of this deforming but non-erosive arthropathy?

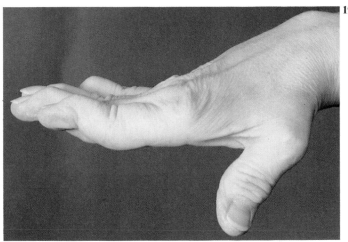

193 (a) What name is given to the sign shown?
(b) Of what rheumatological and connective tissue diseases may this be a feature?
(c) What non-inflammatory disorders may produce similar symptoms?

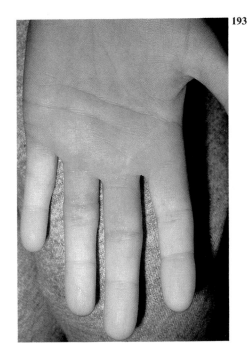

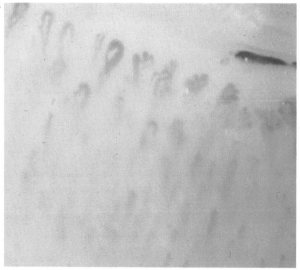

194 The fingernail bed of a patient who presented with dysphagia and admitted to a 5-year history of progressive hand stiffness.

(a) What sign is shown?

(b) What is the probable diagnosis? What other dermatological features should be sought?

(c) How should the dysphagia be investigated? What abnormality would be expected?

(d) What is the cause of the dysphagia? What other gastro-enterological abnormalities may be present in this condition?

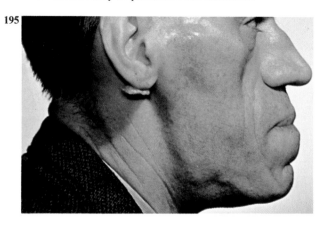

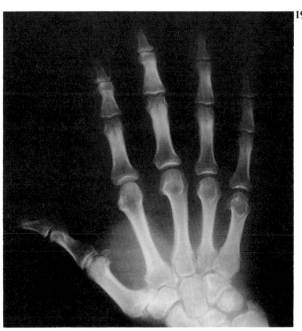

195,196 (a) What abnormalities can be seen in **196**?
(b) What diagnosis is suggested by **195**?
(c) What other radiographic examinations may be used to support this diagnosis?
(d) What form of arthropathy may be associated with this condition?

197 (a) What is this complication of rheumatoid disease?
(b) What causes the blue discoloration of the sclera?

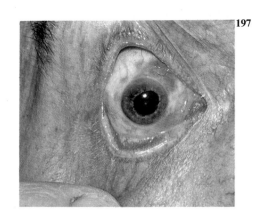

198

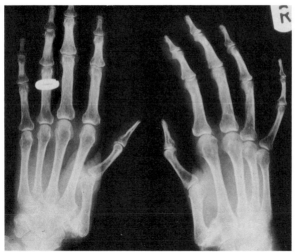

198 The hands of a tall, 46-year-old woman with a history of recurrent dislocation of the patella, elbow and shoulder.
(a) What does the overall appearance of the hands suggest?
(b) The patient is severely visually handicapped. What is the probable cause?
(c) What other skeletal abnormalities occur in this condition?
(d) What secondary complication of joint hypermobility has occurred?

199

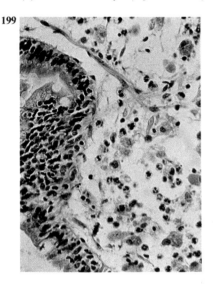

199 A 37-year-old man presented with episodes of abrupt onset synovitis in a migratory pattern involving knees, ankles, wrists and occasionally fingers. He also described weight loss and diarrhoea, and fever associated with the joint symptoms.
(a) What diagnostic feature is demonstrated in this PAS-stained jejunal biopsy?
(b) What is the diagnosis?
(c) What other clinical features may aid diagnosis?
(d) What aetiology does the histological feature suggest? What management should be offered?

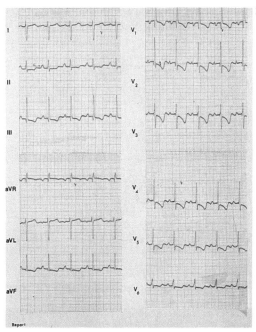

200 A patient with mixed connective tissue disease (predominantly sclerodermatous features with polymyositis) developed limiting exertional breathlessness.

(a) What are the abnormal features on this ECG? What is the underlying problem?

(b) What clinical features should be sought in relation to this abnormality?

(c) What serological finding is typically associated with mixed connective tissue disease?

ANSWERS

1, 2 (a) The loss of joint space at all interphalangeal joints and first carpo-metacarpal joint with osteophyte formation and minimal resultant deformity.
(b) Heberden's nodes (distal) and Bouchard's nodes (proximal). Bony swelling representing osteophyte formation.
(c) Osteoarthrosis. Sparing of the MCP joints, involvement of the DIP joints, lack of osteoporosis, osteophyte formation.

3 (a) Ulnar deviation, subluxation at the MCP joints and subcutaneous nodules diagnostic of rheumatoid arthritis. Additional wrist soft tissue swelling is less specific for rheumatoid disease.
(b) Proximal extensor aspect forearm, and at sites of pressure, eg over Achilles tendon, ischial tuberosity, sacrum and, occasionally, over the helix of the ear.
(c) Solitary pulmonary rheumatoid nodules may require biopsy to exclude carcinoma.
(d) The commonest complication of rheumatoid nodules is ulceration and infection; infected nodules, particularly in the sacral area, may lead to bacteraemia and secondary septic complications.

4 (a) Alopecia and vitiligo.
(b) Systemic lupus erythematosus.

5 (a) Localised rather radio-dense soft tissue swelling over the 2nd to 5th PIP, 3rd DIP and 1st MCP joints, associated with cystic bone lesions, mostly separated from the articular margin.
(b) Gout.
(c) Uricosuric agent (eg probenecid). Urinary urate excretion of more than 700 mg/24 h.
(d) Allopurinol. Commencement of NSAID or low-dose colchicine in addition, as initiation of allopurinol treatment may be associated with acute gout attacks.

6 (a) Sustained elevation of jugular venous pressure in this context suggests tense pericardial effusion or constrictive pericarditis. Cardiac ultrasonography is the most appropriate initial investigation.
(b) High-dose corticosteroids (oral or pulsed intravenously), if no response pericardiocentesis with local corticosteroid injection, if no response pericardectomy.

7, 8 (a) Pseudoxanthoma elasticum.
(b) Angioid streaks (breaks in Bruch's membrane).
(c) Fibrous proliferation and medial calcification of arteries leading to occlusion and rarely ulceration, particularly in the upper limbs. The additional feature of tumoral calcinosis may cause diagnostic confusion with scleroderma.
(d) Two autosomal dominant and two autosomal recessive types have been described.

9 (a) Sickling erythrocytes — sickle cell disease.
(b) Infectious arthritis or acute osteomyelitis — salmonella species are often involved.
(c) Short-lived polyarthralgia during acute sickle crisis, due to subsynovial capillary blockage; avascular necrosis of bone; gout; haemarthrosis (rare).

10 (a) A modified Schöber's test involves marking points 10 cm above and 5 cm below a line joining the 'dimples of Venus' on the sacral promontory. An increase

in separation of less than 5 cm during full forward flexion indicates limited spinal mobility. Finger–floor distance is a simpler indicator, but is less reliable because good hip movement may compensate for back limitation.
(b) Chest expansion (less than 5 cm suggests costo-vertebral involvement); occiput–wall distance (inability to make contact when heel and back are against the wall indicates upper thoracic and cervical limitation).

11, 12 (a) Hyperkeratotic scaling skin lesions; discrete and nummular (guttate) on the legs and coalescing on the feet.
(b) Both have Reiter's syndrome and demonstrate different manifestations of keratoderma blennorrhagia. Pustular psoriasis produces identical clinical and histological features.
(c) Asymmetric joint involvement, enthesopathy, dactylitis, DIP-joint involvement associated with nail changes (uncommon).

13 (a) Soft tissue swelling around the lower portion of the Achilles tendon and its insertion.
(b) Psoriasis with Achilles tendonitis.

14 (a) Spondylolysis due to stress fracture from repeated trauma.
(b) Dysplastic (congenital), degenerative, traumatic, pathological (destructive bone disease) spondylolisthesis.
(c) Compression of nerve roots or cauda equina is more common in degenerative spondylolisthesis, as osteophytic new bone formation tends to narrow the canal. A defect in the pars interarticularis (eg congenital) increases the canal diameter.

15 (a) Trigger finger. Inflammatory change within the flexor tendon sheath results in tendon oedema with 'nodule' formation.
(b) Non-specific tenosynovitis due to occupational trauma. Rest if possible, local steroid injection (note rare possibility of tenolysis), surgical release if simple measures fail.

16 (a) Compression fracture of 11th thoracic vertebra.
(b) Osteoporosis, although osteomalacia should be considered.
(c) Oestrogen, calcium. (Vitamin D and fluoride treatment is controversial.) If osteomalacia is demonstrated by hypocalcaemia, raised alkaline phosphatase, reduced serum 25 hydroxycholecalciferol or bone biopsy vitamin D replacement will be required.

17 (a) Palpebral xanthelasma. Tendon xanthomata. Familial hypercholesterolaemia and familial combined hyperlipidaemia (WHO-types, IIb and IV).
(b) Occasional bone cysts may be identified (WHO-type IV). Erosive changes do not occur.
(c) Weight reduction, iscaloric diet modification (reduce saturated fatty acid intake to less than 10 per cent of energy intake), cholestyramine for hypercholesterolaemia, inositol nicotinate for hypertriglyceridaemia.

18 (a) Psoriasis vulgaris.
(b) Nails, umbilicus, natal cleft, sub-mammary region, scalp.

19–21 (a) Paget's disease.
(b) Osteosarcoma has developed, with bone lysis and spicules of ossification in the tumour soft tissue.
(c) This tumour metastasises early and is not sensitive to chemotherapy. Despite amputation, this patient died within 10 weeks.

22 (a) Two pustules with surrounding erythema.
(b) Gonococcal dermato-arthritis.
(c) Urethral or cervical swab, Gram-stain and culture. (Joint aspirates are usually bacteriologically negative.)

23 (a) Large cystic swelling extending down from the popliteal fossa — Baker's cyst.
(b) Rupture of popliteal cyst usually results in tender, indurated, erythematous swelling of the whole calf. If a gradual leak occurs it may mimic deep-vein thrombosis.
(c) Arthrography will demonstrate leakage of fluid into the calf. Venogram, however, may give false-positive results in Baker's cyst, due to popliteal venous compression.

24 (a) Marked soft tissue swelling in extensor tendon sheath at both wrists (extensor-tenosynovitis). Rheumatoid arthritis.
(b) Extensor tenolysis. Surgical decompression with tendon sheath synovectomy may be safer than corticosteroid injection.

25 (a) Telangiectasia and peri-oral skin puckering. Scleroderma.
(b) The fingernail beds may show dilatation and tortuosity of capillaries (best viewed under a low-power microscope).
(c) The endothelial damage resulting from a circulating protein factor has been implicated as an early component of the 'inflammatory' phase of scleroderma, and endothelial damage may result in the capillary and arteriolar abnormalities demonstrated, and also in local access of circulating proteins acting on fibroblasts enhancing collagen secretion.

26 (a) Inflammatory non-infectious pneumonitis occurs in about 18 per cent of SLE patients at some time.
(b) Bacterial or fungal infection must be excluded (the latter particularly in steroid-treated patients), and pulmonary infarction due to embolism should be considered (patients with the 'lupus anticoagulant' have a high incidence of venous thrombosis).
(c) Pleural effusion in up to 40 per cent of patients.
(d) Forced vital capacity (FVC) is decreased. A ratio of forced expiratory volume in one second (FEV1) to FVC greater than 70 per cent indicates restrictive lung disease, which is the usual pattern. Impaired gas exchange may be demonstrated by reduced carbon monoxide transfer factor and reduced alveolar: arterial oxygen concentration gradient.

27, 28 (a) Joint hypermobility.
(b) Marfan's syndrome, Ehlers–Danlos syndrome, pseudoxanthoma elasticum.
(c) Polyarthralgia without articular abnormality, persistent traumatic inflammatory synovitis with Baker's cyst, recurrent joint dislocation (shoulder and patella), chondromalacia patellae, spinal abnormality including back pain and scoliosis, probable increase of soft tissue lesions (epicondylitis, tendinitis, carpal tunnel syndrome).
(d) Most commonly adolescence and young adulthood (75 per cent before 15 years of age in one study).
(e) Carter and Wilkinson scoring system: (i) hyperextension little fingers beyond 90°; (ii) position of thumb to flexor aspect forearm (illustrated); (iii, iv) hyperextension of elbows and knees beyond 10°; (v) forward flexion of trunk with legs straight with palms resting flat on floor. One point for each item, total 9.

29 (a) Rheumatoid pleural effusions are commonly asymptomatic and detected incidentally, though they may present as pleurisy, breathlessness if severe, and in association with pericarditis.
(b) Males are affected more commonly than females.
(c) Tuberculosis and tumour. No, although a very low glucose associated with a high rheumatoid factor and high protein is suggestive of rheumatoid effusion.

30 (a) Swelling over the carpal tunnel, anterior aspect wrist. Some thenar eminence wasting is also present.
(b) Median nerve compression. Nerve conduction studies.
(c) Immobilisation in a simple splint, injection with corticosteroids, surgical release.

31 (a) Clubbing.
(b) Hypertrophic pulmonary osteoarthropathy. Intrathoracic tumours (eg bronchial, pleural, but very rarely metastases), suppurative intrathoracic conditions (bronchiectasis, lung abscess, empyema), tuberculosis, cystic fibrosis, mediastinal Hodgkin's lymphoma.
(c) Removal of a primary carcinoma; if inoperable, intrathoracic vagotomy.

32, 33 (a) Osteoarthrosis (secondary).
(b) Childhood rickets.

34 (a) Paget's disease (osteitis deformans).
(b) Osteoarthritis right hip with degenerative change symphysis pubis.
(c) Pelvic deformity causing difficult acetabular replacement, and Pagetic bone consistency brittle and hard.

35 (a) Pyoderma gangrenosum.
(b) The skin ulceration has an irregular outline with a ragged bluish-red overhanging edge and an oedematous red crater with a necrotic base.
(c) Vasculitic damage, with resultant granulating ulceration.

36, 37 (a) Luminal narrowing by oedematus intima, histiocytic and lymphocytic infiltrate and multinucleate giant cells.
(b) Giant-cell arteritis involves medium-sized and large arteries typically in the cranial distribution from, and including, the aorta. The temporal artery is clinically and surgically easily accessible.
(c) Systemic features include polymyalgia rheumatica, fever, weight loss and malaise, and anaemia and abnormal liver function tests (particularly raised alkaline phosphatase) may be present. Cerebral and retinal infarction may occur. The ESR is almost invariably markedly elevated. High-dose oral prednisolone commencing at 60 mg daily with reduction in dosage guided by normalisation of the ESR and symptoms.

38 (a) Wegener's granulomatosis.
(b) Glomerulonephritis with hypertension and renal failure.
(c) Alkylating agents such as cyclophosphamide.

39 (a) Scleroderma (progressive systemic sclerosis). An early oedematous phase (with pitting oedema of hands and possibly forearms, legs and face), followed by dermal thickening with skin tightness. An atrophic phase with contracture may follow.
(b) Depigmentation is apparent. Either pigmentation or speckled depigmentation may be observed.

40 (a) Grey/bronze pigmentation. Haemochromatosis.
(b) Calcium pyrophosphate deposition with resultant degenerative arthropathy. Chondrocalcinosis.
(c) Marked elevation in serum iron (> 30 μmol/l (175 μg/100 ml)) and 75–100 per cent transferrin saturation. Liver biopsy is the definitive test.
(d) Arthropathy as for osteoarthrosis. Weekly or twice-weekly phlebotomy of 500 ml — supportive therapy for hepatic and cardiac failure and diabetes.

41 (a) Scleritis.
(b) Rheumatoid arthritis.
(c) Dry, gritty eyes due to keratoconjunctivitis sicca (in Sjögren's syndrome).

42 (a) Acute sarcoidosis (hilar lymphadenopathy is demonstrated).
(b) Erythema nodosum.
(c) Hyperglobulinaemia and anergy (defective delayed hypersensitivity response to skin antigen testing). Rheumatoid factor is sometimes positive.

43 (a) Nail dystrophy with onycholysis and adjacent DIP-joint involvement.
(b) Nail dystrophy is more common in psoriatic patients with arthritis (80 per cent) than those without (20 per cent), and is associated with local DIP-joint involvement.
(c) Trauma, in psoriatic arthritis.

44 (a) Dry tongue. Xerostomia due to Sjögren's syndrome.
(b) Lachrymal (keratoconjunctivitis sicca), vaginal (may cause dyspareunia), occasionally bronchial.
(c) Labial salivary gland biopsy under local anaesthetic.

45, 46 (a) Arthritis mutilans with 'pencil in cup' deformity.
(b) Rheumatoid arthritis, psoriatic arthritis.
(c) 'Main en lorgnette', or opera-glass hand, because osteolytic bone loss results in telescoping of the fingers.

47, 48 (a) Anti-nuclear antibody.
(b) A large number of nuclear proteins have been shown to complex with circulating antibodies, explaining the lack of specificity of this test for SLE. These include DNA, nuclear ribonuclear protein (n-RNP), SM, nuclear histone and nuclear RNA. Different patterns of fluorescence occur depending on antigen distribution.
(c) Homogeneous and nucleolar patterns. Nucleolar pattern is associated with systemic sclerosis.

49 (a) Knee joint effusion with massive fluid accumulation in suprapatellar bursa.
(b) Acute post-dysenteric (reactive) synovitis. Salmonella, shigella, yersinia, and campylobacter species have all been implicated. Inflammatory bowel disease should be considered.

50 (a) Romanus lesions.
(b) Inflammation in the region of the annulus fibrosus is associated with adjacent vertebral osteitis. Healing with ossification leads to bridging syndesmophytes.
(c) Squaring of the anterior aspect of the vertebrae.

51 (a) Epiphyseal overgrowth, most apparent in the tibia.
(b) Leg length discrepancy (right leg overgrowth) may result in abnormal gait and

compensatory scoliosis. Suppression of inflammation may include intra-articular steroids, and a heel-raise may be needed.

(c) Pauciarticular juvenile chronic arthritis. Chronic iridocyclitis (usually initially asymptomatic), occurs in 10–50 per cent of patients, and 6-monthly slit-lamp examinations should be performed.

52 Premature fusion of 4th metacarpal epyphysis. There is also a periosteal reaction over the distal ulnar aspect of this bone.

53 (a) Very heavy iron staining.
(b) Serum iron falls very quickly after onset of acute or chronic inflammation, and ferritin is synthesised by cells of the reticuloendothelial system as part of the 'acute phase response'.
(c) Bone marrow examination is the only reliable test.

54 (a) Marked osteoporosis with multiple compression fractures of the thoracic vertebrae ('vertebra plana').
(b) Corticosteroid administration.
(c) Active systemic juvenile arthritis (Still's disease) is usually associated with marked slowing or virtual cessation of growth. Also, he has lost vertical height and corticosteroids will impair linear growth.
(d) Single daily morning dose or preferably alternate-day dosage. Breakthrough fever is best treated with indomethacin, aspirin or tolmetin.

55 (a) Circinate balanitis.
(b) Reiter's syndrome.
(c) Urethritis, prostatitis (with occasional abscess formation), haemorrhagic cystitis, rarely ureteric obstruction with hydronephrosis.

56 (a) Gouty tophi on the ear.
(b) Toes, forefeet, hands, ulnar border of the forearm, olecranon bursa, Achilles tendon.
(c) Hyperlipidaemia (WHO-type 2A — familial hypercholesterolaemia), multicentric reticulohistiocytosis.

57 (a) Mucosal ulceration with surrounding erythema and induration. Behçet's syndrome.
(b) CNS involvement and major blood vessel occlusion.
(c) There are no tests diagnostic for Behçet's syndrome. Evidence of an acute inflammatory response, polyclonal immunoglobulin increase and mild to moderate anaemia are similar to other chronic inflammatory disorders. The 'pathergy' test (a pustule with surrounding erythema develops 24 h after sterile pin-prick of the skin) appears to be less common in British than in Turkish cases.

58 (a) Periorbital oedema.
(b) Dermatomyositis. Nephrotic syndrome due to systemic lupus erythematosus with glomerulonephritis.
(c) Her CPK was grossly elevated, and muscle biopsy confirmed inflammatory myositis. DNA binding (anti-DNA antibody) was normal, making SLE unlikely.

59, 60 (a) Dupuytren's contracture and knuckle pads of Garrod.
(b) None. It is a localised sclerosis, but may be associated with Peyronie's disease and plantar fibromatosis, and in some cases has a strong familial tendency.

61, 62 (a) Henoch–Schönlein purpura.
(b) Non-thrombocytopenic leucocytoclastic vasculitis.
(c) Gastro-intestinal involvement with abdominal pain and occasional gastro-intestinal haemorrhage, mesenteric infarction, and intussusception in young children. Glomerulonephritis (progressive renal insufficiency is uncommon).
(d) Upper respiratory infection.
(e) Over 90 per cent of patients have a short self-limiting course for which simple symptomatic treatments are sufficient. Corticosteroids may be used for relapsing or persistent involvement, although there is little evidence that they prevent renal impairment.

63, 64 (a) Those of central necrosis, palisading elongated connective tissue cells (histiocytes) radiating out to enveloping chronic inflammatory granulation tissue are typical of a rheumatoid nodule, pathognomonic for rheumatoid arthritis.
(b) Sclera, lungs and pleura, heart, vocal cords.
(c) Gouty tophi, xanthoma in hyperlipidaemia, multi-centric reticulohistiocytosis.

65, 66 (a) Distal IP joint involvement, absence of wrist involvement and the large size of the dorsal hand swelling.
(b) Gout.
(c) Polarised-light microscopy of the oelecronon bursa discharge will show needle-shaped, strongly negatively birefringent crystals.
(d) Tophaceous gout will progress if untreated, with bone destruction and accumulation of unsightly discharging tophi. Lowering serum uric acid (usually with allopurinol, possibly a uricosuric agent) allows gradual mobilisation and resolution of deposits.

67 (a) Erythema nodosum.
(b) Erythema nodosum from any cause may be associated with arthralgia or frank synovitis. Therefore, acute sarcoidosis, tuberculosis, Crohn's disease, post-streptococcal or post-sulphonamide EN must all be considered.
(c) Symptoms and signs of eye inflammation and lymphadenopathy may indicate acute sarcoidosis; respiratory symptoms with sweats and weight loss may suggest tuberculosis; abdominal pain and/or diarrhoea or abdominal mass for Crohn's disease, or recent sore throat or antibiotic exposure.
(d) Chest X-ray (hilar lymphadenopathy in sarcoid, pneumonitis in tuberculosis), serial antistreptolysin–O titre, barium contrast studies or abdominal ultrasonography if gastro-intestinal symptoms suggest Crohn's disease.

68 Ruptured long head of biceps.

69, 70 (a) Calcinosis tip right index finger in the photograph, and also in the middle finger and flexor aspect of the thumb in the X-ray.
(b) Sclerodactyly, possibly skin thickening on the face, telangiectases around the mouth and dorsal hands, dilated capillaries at the nail beds.
(c) As well as the palmar aspects of the terminal phalanges and the MCP joint of the thumb, the extensor surface of the forearms, the olecranon bursa and prepatellar area may be involved.
(d) CREST syndrome (calcinosis, Raynaud's phenomenon, oesophageal abnormality, sclerodactyly, telangiectasia). Systemic sclerosis (scleroderma).

71, 72 (a) Rheumatoid arthritis. MCP joint swelling and subluxation with ulnar

deformity; fixed flexion 1st MCP joint.
(b) Swan-neck deformity.
(c) Swanson type MCP prosthesis.

73 (a) Hyperplasia of synovial lining cells, lymphocytic infiltrate with dense lymphocytic aggregate at the top left-hand corner. Special staining with methyl-green/pyronin (not shown here) would demonstrate numerous plasma cells.
(b) Strongly HLA-DR positive cells of macrophage lineage (dendritic or antigen-presenting cells) associated with excess of t-helper lymphocytes (OKT4 positive) over t-suppresser lymphocytes (OKT8 positive), and also surface immunoglobulin bearing B-lymphocytes.
(c) Interleukin-1 (lymphocyte activating factor) is macrophage-derived and potentiates lymphocyte activation and antigen priming. Interleukin-2 (t-cell growth factor) is T-lymphocyte-derived and it potentiates T-lymphocyte proliferation. Other locally produced factors include interferon-gamma, B-cell growth factor.

74 (a) Rheumatoid erosions occur first where hypertrophied synovium is limited by joint capsule insertion; inflammatory pannus will be invading the eroded cartilage and bone.
(b) Although temporary improvement in pain and swelling occurs, its present use is limited to the knees, to tendon decompression in the hands and wrists, and in conjunction with other procedures, such as radial head excision at the elbow.

75 (a) Rheumatoid nodules.
(b) Reiter's syndrome, ankylosing spondylitis, rheumatoid arthritis, hyperlipid-aemia.

76 (a) Infiltration of retina around lower nasal vessel, associated with localised retinal haemorrhage.
(b) Systemic lupus erythematosus. Retinal vasculitis (here in severe form) reflects the diffuse cerebral small vessel inflammatory vasculopathy responsible for the organic brain syndrome.
(c) Positive anti-nuclear antibody with antibody to double-stranded DNA, evidence of complement consumption, leukopenia and/or thrombocytopenia. CSF abnormalities (increased protein, occasional pleocytosis) and EEG abnormalities have been reported.

77, 78 (a) A renal parenchymal mass penetrating the renal cortex with tumour circulation — renal carcinoma.
(b) Infiltration of muscle fibres with lymphocytes and histiocytes, with evidence of fibre necrosis and fragmentation. Acute myositis.
(c) Nephrectomy should be performed. In the absence of secondary spread the myositis may regress. High-dose oral prednisolone supplemented by methotrexate if necessary.

79 (a) Psoriatic arthropathy. DIP involvement (also deformity and swelling of left 4th PIP joint).
(b) Pain, loss of thumb mobility and ability to oppose, fixed MCP-subluxation, constrictive flexor tendon involvement.

80 (a) Bruising due to thrombocytopoenia.
(b) Platelet count below 100,000 is reported in up to 20 per cent of routine clinical surveys, though profound thrombocytopoenia with bleeding is much rarer. If associated with *neutropenia* the prognosis is more serious.

(c) Recent evidence suggests isolated thrombocytopoenia is usually due to immune peripheral platelet destruction, although severe pancytopoenia (very rarely fatal) appears to reflect bone marrow suppression. Stopping penicillamine usually results in rise in platelet count within 10 days. Corticosteroids are beneficial, and platelet infusions are rarely required.

(d) Regular (fortnightly or monthly) platelet count. If a downward trend is observed, even within the normal range, the drug should be stopped, with reintroduction at a lower dosage when recovered.

81 (a) Incomplete cortical interruption without displacement. Looser's zone, or 'pseudofracture'.

(b) Osteomalacia. Axillary margins of scapulae, ribs, superior and inferior pubic rami, inner proximal femora, posterior margins proximal ulnae. They are often symmetrical.

(c) Serum calcium will be reduced, alkaline phosphatase normal or elevated, 25-hydroxycholecalciferol will be reduced. Xylose absorption and jejunal biopsy may show evidence of malabsorption. Urine analysis may show increase of tubular phosphate loss or tubular acidosis.

82 (a) 'Squaring' of the base of the thumb. Heberden's nodes with 2nd DIP deformity.

(b) Degenerative change in the 1st carpo-metacarpal joint. Loss of thumb abduction.

(c) Generalised osteoarthrosis.

83, 84 Arachnodactyly (long thumb protruding beyond narrow palm).

(b) Arm-span greater than height. (The bruising is related to vessel puncture during cardiac investigation.)

(c) Marfan's syndrome.

(d) Both aortic regurgitation and dissecting aneurysm may occur; mitral regurgitation is occasionally functionally significant.

85 (a) Infarction of the nail bed due to small vessel vasculitis.

(b) Subcutaneous rheumatoid nodules most commonly found on the extensor surface of the forearms, over the fingers and at pressure sites, such as the sacrum or Achilles tendon; vasculitic ulcers on the shins (rarely pyoderma gangrenosum); palpable vasculitic purpura may occur around the buttocks.

86 (a) Soft tissue opacity, representing tumorous calcinosis.

(b) Hyperphosphataemia. Phosphate-binding drugs and effective dialysis.

(c) Eyes, arteries, in periarticular capsule and tendons of large and small joints, and in cartilage. Deposits may be single or multiple, and are often multiloculated.

(d) Calcific tendinitis (eg supraspinatus tendon), pseudo-gout.

87 (a) A bone fragment is separated from the medial femoral condyle, though not displaced — osteochondritis dissecans.

(b) With this occupation the cause is probably traumatic, although anomalous ossification and locally deficient blood supply have been implicated in some patients. Conservative treatment, unless loose body demands removal or fixation.

(c) The capitellum of the elbow, the talus of the ankle, the hip, the metatarsal heads.

88 (a) Dilated temporal artery. Local tenderness and absence of pulsation.

(b) Visual disturbance, including clouding, transient loss of vision, field defect;

symptoms of transient cerebral ischaemia; claudication of the jaw; morning stiffness; functional limitation of standing up or climbing stairs.
(c) Immediate administration of high-dose oral corticosteroids (30–60 mg daily) after taking blood for ESR. This may be gradually reduced after control of symptoms and fall in ESR.

89 (a) Asymmetrical osteophyte formation and sclerosis adjacent to the inter-vertebral discs.
(b) Degenerative spinal arthropathy. Advanced asymmetrical changes probably result from scoliosis.
(c) Syndesmophytes grow vertically by ossification of the annulus fibrosus with eventual bony bridging (ankylosis). Osteophytes develop laterally ('spreading the load') without ankylosing.

90 (a) Desquamation over the 1st MTP joint; some residual erythema.
(b) Gout (classical podagra).
(c) No regular medication. A supply of effective NSAID such as indomethacin for future attack should be provided. Indications for regular medication such as allo-purinol are frequent acute attacks (more often than every 3 months), development of tophi, nephrolithiasis or renal function impairment.

91 (a) Bridging syndesmophyte formation with ankylosis between lumbar vertebrae ('bamboo spine'), sacro-iliac joint fusion, ossification of the posterior spinal liga-ment.
(b) Ankylosing spondylitis.

92 (a) Septic arthritis.
(b) *Staphylococcus aureus.*
(c) Full-dose intravenous anti-staphylococcal antibiotic for at least 2 weeks, followed by oral antibodies to a total of 6 weeks.
(d) Surgical drainage.

93 (a) Erosive sacro-iliitis on the right.
(b) Urethritis and prostatitis may both occur in Reiter's syndrome and less commonly in ankylosing spondylitis, and may result in microscopic haematuria.

94 (a) Dermatitis is the commonest side-effect of gold (myocrisin) treatment. Most rashes are pruritic, 30 per cent resemble lichen planus and 10 per cent resemble pityriasis rosea (as in this case). Pruritus and rash occur commonly during penicilla-mine treatment. Pemphigoid bullous lesions also occur.
(b) Cessation of gold injections resulting in disappearance of the rash may be followed by cautious re-introduction after a few weeks, often without loss of disease control.

95, 96 (a) Myeloma (plasmacytoma or multiple myeloma). Skull, pelvis, ribs.
(b) Trinucleate (neoplastic) plasma cell.
(c) Secondary amyloidosis.
(d) Evidence of widespread marrow replacement (anaemia, leukopoenia, thrombo-cytopoenia, leuko-erythroblastic blood film), reduction of other immunoglobin levels (immunoparesis), bone lysis.
(e) Avoid dehydration — intravenous urography may precipitate acute renal failure.

97, 98 (a) Paget's disease.
(b) Calcitonin, diphosphonates.
(c) Serum alkaline phosphatase and urinary hydroxyproline excretion.
(d) Not normally, but it may occur during immobilisation.

99 (a) Calcaneal spur with rather indistinct and irregular outline.
(b) Reiter's syndrome. Conjunctivitis is typical, iritis occurs in 5–10 per cent of patients. Retinitis with macular oedema, and optic neuritis have rarely been reported.

100, 101 (a) Diffuse increase in interstitial lung markings, tending to spare the upper zones. By the second radiograph the infiltrate is much denser in patches with some almost discrete nodules. The heart size has also increased.
(b) Dust exposure has led to pneumoconiosis.
(c) Caplan's syndrome.

102, 103 (a) Livedo reticularis with two localised necrotic lesions on the calf; palpable purpura.
(b) Rheumatoid vasculitis. Circulating immune complexes with evidence of complement consumption (absent in uncomplicated rheumatoid arthritis).
(c) Vasculitis appears to be involved in pathogenesis of rheumatoid nodules, peripheral neuropathy, mononeuritis multiplex (rare), scleritis and scleromalacia perforans, and pleuropericardial involvement.

104 (a) Thermography of the hands. The hand on the left shows cold fingers, suggesting marked reduction of blood flow to the fingers. This is Raynaud's phenomenon.
(b) Monitoring of joint activity in inflammatory arthritis. Results are affected by soft tissue thickness, and it gives poor comparative data between patients. Deep-sited joints such as the hip cannot be adequately measured, results depend critically on ambient conditions, measurement is time-consuming.

105 (a) Scleroderma.
(b) Vasculitis. Digital infarction is the commonest necrotising manifestation. Renal vessel involvement is characterised by intimal hyperplasia and fibrinoid necrosis ('nephrosclerosis'), not with inflammatory cell infiltrate.
(c) Pulmonary hypertension with right heart failure, cardiac arrhythmias including complete heart block, pericarditis, cardiac failure due to myocardial fibrosis.

106 (a) Rickets.
(b) Low serum calcium and phosphate, raised alkaline phosphatase, reduced 25-hydroxycholecalciferol, raised serum parathyroid hormone.
(c) Therapeutic trial of vitamin D.

107 (a) Exposure of the metatarsal head due to metatarso-phalangeal subluxation resulting in callous formation.
(b) Rheumatoid arthritis.
(c) Support of the metatarsal shafts relieves pressure during walking. An external metatarsal bar under the sole usually provides better relief than a metatarsal support insole.

108 (a) Felty's syndrome (localised shin pigmentation is also quite common in active rheumatoid disease without neutropenia).
(b) Lithium carbonate is a simple means of improving white cell count in some patients; control of disease activity using gold, penicillamine, or even cyclophosphamide has been successful, though very close monitoring is required; the late results of splenectomy are disappointing, and perioperative mortality is high.
(c) Ulceration of the lower leg.

109 (a) Legg–Perthes disease.
(b) Ideopathic osteonecrosis (avascular necrosis) of the proximal femoral epiphysis.

(c) Young males (average age 7 years).
(d) Relief from weight-bearing (ambulation is possible using a Snyder sling), and maintenance of the femoral head within the acetabulum (plaster immobilisation and/or surgery may rarely be required).

110 (a) Nephrotic syndrome due to secondary amyloid deposition.
(b) Alkylating agents, specifically chlorambucil, have been recommended for progressive secondary amyloidosis with renal involvement, and arrest of the inflammatory process has been associated with resolution of the disorder. Sterility is almost universal after as little as 3 months of continuous treatment; treatment over several years may result in the late development of leukaemia.
(c) Rectal biopsy, needle aspiration biopsy of abdominal wall fat.

111 (a) Calcific opacity in the medial and lateral meniscus.
(b) They are probably unrelated. Asymptomatic chondrocalcinosis has been demonstrated in up to 27 per cent of the elderly population. Finger joint involvement is not typical of calcium pyrophosphate deposition disease.

112 (a) Partial obliteration of C3/4 neural foramen.
(b) Osteophyte formation in the apophyseal joint.
(c) No intervention in the absence of symptoms. Pain and paraesthesiae may respond to intermittent cervical collar. Surgical decompression should be considered only if progressive motor weakness develops.

113 (a) New bone formation at muscle–tendon–bone junctions — a form of enthesopathy.
(b) Fusion of the sacro-iliac joints (there is also some narrowing and irregularity of the left hip joint with early flattening of the femoral head). Ankylosing spondylitis.

114 (a) Wasting of the thenar eminence.
(b) Median nerve compression.
(c) Hypothyroidism, diabetes mellitus, acromegaly (rare).

115 (a) Infectious arthritis, osteomyelitis, haemarthrosis. (Joint involvement in systemic JCA is usually polyarticular.)
(b) Any source of infection? Any observed bleeding tendency following lacerations/trauma? Any family history of bleeding tendency?
(c) Haemophilia.
(d) Marked overgrowth of the radial head, moderate cartilage loss and early degenerative change.

116 (a) Extensive loss of haustral pattern of the descending colon with irregular mucosal patterns suggesting ulceration. Ulcerative colitis.
(b) Yes: 66–75 per cent of patients with colitic arthritis show such a relationship.
(c) Erythema nodosum. Acute anterior uveitis, pyoderma gangrenosum.
(d) Colonic bowel wall damage may permit exposure of colonic bacterial or ingested antigen to the sytemic circulation, producing immune complexes which may mediate systemic damage, or antibodies which may cross-react with skin, eye or blood vessel antigens.

117 (a) Swelling of the index finger.
(b) Dactylitis typically occurs in psoriatic arthritis and Reiter's syndrome.
(c) Joint and tendon sheath synovium, periosteum. A periosteal reaction is sometimes observed.

118 (a) Muscle fibre atrophy, marked fibrosis, mild mononuclear cell infiltrate.

(b) Fibrosis and a relatively mild mononuclear cell infiltrate indicate that weakness is primarily due to established muscle destruction, and the risks of powerful immunosuppressive agents are probably not justified.

119 (a) Infective arthritis or crystal arthritis, specifically pseudo-gout.

(b) Joint aspiration, radiography. (Serum uric acid, calcium, alkaline phosphatase may all provide supportive information.)

(c) Calcium pyrophosphate is responsible for chondrocalcinosis in cases of pseudo-gout.

(d) Weakly positively birefringent rhomboid microcrystals, commonly intra-cellular.

(e) The knees. Chondrocalcinosis may be observed in the knees (articular hyaline cartilage and meniscal fibrocartilage), the wrists and the symphysis pubis.

120 (a) Herpes zoster infection (shingles).

(b) Electron-microscopy of fresh vesicle fluid.

(c) Sytemic antiviral treatment, eg intravenous Acyclovir (dissemination of viral infection is a potential risk in any immunosuppressed patient).

121, 122 (a) Loss of peristalsis in the oesophagus. Dysphagia and reflux oesophagitis due to functional interruption of the cardiac sphincter.

(b) Wide-mounted diverticulae on the antimesenteric border of the transverse and descending colon. Intestinal perforation, obstruction, volvulus and pneumatosis intestinalis are rare complications.

(c) Progressive systemic sclerosis (scleroderma).

(d) Bloating, abdominal cramps and episodic diarrhoea or constipation reflect small intestinal hypomotility resulting in bacterial overgrowth and fat malabsorption. Broad-spectrum antibiotic treatment often improves these symptoms.

123 Reiter's syndrome. Keratoderma blenorrhagica (although usually confined to the soles of the feet, it may affect all the digits, as shown, and extend to the limbs and trunk).

124 (a) Systemic onset of juvenile arthritis. Arthropathy associated with viral infection (rubella, infectious mononucleosis), Henoch–Schönlein purpura, acute leukaemia.

(b) Lymphadenopathy, hepatosplenomegaly, pleuro-pulmonary involvement and pericarditis, rarely myocarditis.

(c) Reduction in linear growth, osteoporosis with compression spinal fracture, truncal obesity, loss of muscle bulk and strength, cataract. NSAID such as aspirin and indomethacin effectively control fever in many patients. Steroid use should be restricted for serious systemic complications or disabling arthritis, and given in alternate-day dosage.

125 (a) Myocrisin and D-penicillamine.

(b) White blood cell count and platelet count, and urine for protein before every myocrisin injection and monthly following commencement of penicillamine.

126 (a) Sarcoidosis.

(b) Superficial involvement is demonstrated (episcleritis). Anterior uveitis is more typical (iris and ciliary body).

(c) Post-streptococcal or occasionally post-viral reactive synovitis associated with erythema nodosum. (Tuberculosis is not a cause of acute joint symptoms, but should be considered in any case of erythema nodosum.)

(d) Widespread lymphadenopathy including bilateral hilar lymphadenopathy would support a diagnosis of acute sarcoidosis.

127 (a) A chronic synovial lesion producing bleeding in the absence of a generalised bleeding tendency, suggesting pigmented villonodular synovitis.
(b) The synovium in pigmented villonodular synovitis is red-brown, markedly thickened, and matted masses of villous projections and folds coalesce to produce sessile or pedunculated nodules.
(c) It occurs in young adults, and 80 per cent present with unilateral knee involvement.
(d) Total surgical synovectomy.

128 (a) Elongated crystals which are refractile in certain axes but not in others.
(b) Birefringence is the variation in the velocity of light passing through an ordered structure in different directions. Urate crystals (which these are) are needle-shaped, and strongly birefringent. The birefringence disappears (extinction angle) when their long axis is parallel to that of the crossed polariser. The extinction angle for the rhomboid crystals of calcium pyrophosphate is 20–30°.

129 (a) Metacarpal metaphyseal lysis with periosteal new bone formation on metacarpal shafts.
(b) Acute leukaemia. Bone marrow aspiration.
(c) Additive or migratory polyarticular involvement from synovial infiltration (mainly knees, shoulders and ankles) aggravated during blast crisis. Secondary gout. Occasionally septic arthritis may be seen.

130 (a) Puffy swelling of the dorsum of the hand and fingers with nail discolouration. Shoulder–hand syndrome.
(b) Skin atrophy with scaling and desquamation, loss of hair or hypertrichosis. The extremity may be cool and pale, or warm and erythematous, reflecting vasomotor instability.
(c) Patchy or mottled osteoporosis; fine-detail radiography may show sub-periosteal, endosteal and sub-chondral resorption, which may cause cortical breaks or fragmentation resembling rheumatoid erosive disease.
(d) Hemiplegia, herpes zoster (shingles) with post-herpetic neuralgia, epilepsy, rarely pulmonary tuberculosis.

131 (a) Concentric rings of periarteriolar fibrosis with 'onion skin' appearance. Systemic lupus erythematosus.
(b) It is thought to be the end-stage of earlier focal arteritis.

132 (a) Fibrosing alveolitis — cryptogenic (30 per cent have significant rheumatoid factor) or associated with rheumatoid disease or SLE.
(b) Corticosteroids may be used in the early stages. Immunosuppressive regimes, including cyclophosphamide, have been used.

133 (a) Erosive changes in both sacro-iliac joints, with apparent joint widening and marginal sclerosis.
(b) Post-dysenteric Reiter's syndrome. Ankylosing spondylitis and spondylitis associated with inflammatory bowel disease.
(c) Planter fasciitis. Local corticosteroid injection.

134 (a) Systemic lupus erythematosus.
(b) Antinuclear factor with DNA binding, urine analysis for protein, full blood count for leukopenia and/or thrombocytopenia.
(c) Use ultraviolet light screening creams during sun-exposure.

135 (a) Indentation of the contrast column due to posterolateral protrusion of L5/S1 disc, with obstruction of the nerve root sheath on the right.
(b) Strict supine rest (the advantage of traction is probably simply that it enforces rest) and adequate analgesia.
(c) Loss of motor power in affected nerve root, impaired bladder or bowel control, severe and unremitting pain.

136 (a) Steroid-induced purpura.
(b) Reduction in structural connective tissue proteins supporting small vessel walls. Similar impairment in structural protein synthesis in bone results in osteoporosis.

137 (a) Localised conjunctival injection with small rheumatoid nodule by lateral end lower lid.
(b) Perforation of the globe at the site of the rheumatoid nodule.

138 (a) Protrusio acetabuli.
(b) Long-standing rheumatoid arthritis with hip involvement. Paget's disease, osteomalacia.
(c) Placement of the acetabular component of a total hip replacement may be technically difficult.

139 (a) Digital vasculitis, resulting in digital gangrene.
(b) Corticosteroids, cyclophosphamide (including pulsed intravenous cyclophosphamide), prostacyclin (prostaglandin I_2) infusion.

140 (a) Ciliary injection, hypopyon level and adhesions between iris and lens (synechiae).
(b) Acute anterior uveitis.
(c) Seronegative spondyloarthrophies, specifically ankylosing spondylitis. Sacroilliac joint X-ray showing erosion, sclerosis or ankylosis.

141 (a) Interruption on cortex right femoral head, with loss of contour. Avascular necrosis.
(b) Alcoholism, corticosteroids (including Cushing's syndrome), hyperlipidaemia, haemoglobinopathy, decompression (Caisson disease). Serum lipids.
(c) Progression to secondary osteoarthritis and probable need for total hip replacement within 10 years.

142 (a) Sclerotic lumbar vertebra.
(b) Carcinoma of the prostate, Paget's disease.
(c) Serum acid phosphatase.
(d) It will not help to differentiate, but may indicate other sites of involvement.

143 (a) Swan-neck deformity (right 3rd, 4th, 5th fingers), boutonnière (right 2nd finger) and 'Z' deformity (thumb).
(b) DIP-joint involvement most evident in the left hand.

144 (a) Popliteal (Baker's) cyst.
(b) It may confirm meniscus and cruciate ligament damage in the knee, and the presence of loose bodies, but is mainly superseded by arthroscopy for intra-articular mechanical derangement.

145 (a) A discrete nodule in the left lung. (Lateral view showed this to be associated with the oblique fissure.)

(b) Solitary rheumatoid nodule, bronchogenic carcinoma, possible alveolar cell carcinoma.
(c) Bronchoscopy with open-lung biopsy if necessary. In this case biopsy demonstrated rheumatoid nodule.

146 (a) Micrognathia.
(b) Cervical spine involvement.
(c) Major difficulty may be experienced in endotracheal intubation.

147, 148 (a) Thickening of the Achilles tendon insertion suggesting an inflammatory lesion (Achilles tendonitis/enthesopathy), with scar over medial malleolus.
(b) Erosion of Achilles tendon insertion.
(c) Reiter's syndrome, possibly psoriatic arthropathy, or other seronegative spondylarthropathy (eg ankylosing spondylitis). Urethral discharge, conjunctivitis, skin rash (soles of the feet, nail beds as in keratoderma blenorrhagica, or typical psoriatic sites). Occupational or sporting trauma may produce an inflammatory tendinitis, but without erosion.
(d) If active urethritis is present, tetracycline or equivalent should be prescribed; there is no evidence that it reduces Reiter's arthritis. If traumatic, rest is the most appropriate therapy. Local injection of corticosteroids may be associated with Achilles tendon rupture, and should be used with great caution.

149 (a) Opacity of the cornea. Band keratopathy.
(b) Pauciarticular juvenile chronic arthritis.
(c) Slit-lamp examination of all children with pauciarticular arthritis at regular intervals to detect asymptomatic chronic anterior uveitis.

150 (a) Areas of depigmentation and some enhanced pigmentation. Some localised skin ulceration.
(b) Scleroderma.
(c) Evidence of restrictive lung defect should be sought, specifically vital capacity. Evidence of progressive restriction or impairment of gas exchange (eg carbon monoxide transfer factor) indicates progressive fibrosis.
(d) None is proven to be effective. Corticosteroids, penicillamine and immunosuppressive regimes have all been recommended.

151 (a) Low-voltage complexes suggest pericardial effusion. Ventricular extrasystoles are also present.
(b) Elevated JVP, enlarged liver, pulsus paradoxus (fall of more than 10 mmHg in systolic blood pressure on inspiration).
(c) Hypothyroidism.

152 (a) Lymphoid cells (lymphocytes and plasma cells) with a central myoepithelial cell island.
(b) Sjögren's syndrome associated with rheumatoid arthritis. Keratoconjunctivitis sicca and xerostomia.
(c) Respiratory tract (nasal and bronchial mucosa), gastro-intestinal tract (dysphagia, achlorhydria, pancreatic and hepatobiliary involvement), kidney (renal tubular defects such as nephrogenic diabetes insipidus, acidosis).
(d) Lymphoreticular malignancy (typically reticulum cell sarcoma and primitive undifferentiated lymphoma).

153 (a) Fragmentation of the tibial tuberosity at the patellar tendon with some separation of the ossification centre. Osgood–Schlatter disease.
(b) Age 11–15 years. Sporting activity and rapid growth are both associated. The condition is usually unilateral.

154 Fusion of apophyseal joints of all cervical vertebrae. This occurs much more commonly in juvenile onset inflammatory arthritis than in adult rheumatoid arthritis.

155, 156 (a) Spondylitis associated with psoriasis.
(b) Bridging syndesmophytes between 2nd and 3rd, and 3rd and 4th vertebrae, with ankylosis of apophyseal joints of 2nd and 3rd vertebrae.
(c) Psoriatic spondylitis. Predominant DIP joint involvement with nail lesions (5–16 per cent of psoriatic arthritis), arthritis mutilans (5 per cent), symmetrical polyarthritis resembling rheumatoid arthritis (15 per cent), mono- or asymmetrical oligo-articular arthritis with scattered DIP, PIP and MP joint involvement (70 per cent).

157 (a) Fragmentation and resorption of the terminal phalangeal tufts, and early calcinosis around the DIP-joints.
(b) Bone resorption occurs occasionally in the middle phalanx, and rarely in the distal radius and ulna, at the acromioclavicular joint, at the angle of the mandible and in the ribs (resulting in 'rib notching').

158, 159 (a) Relapsing polychondritis.
(b) Labyrinthine damage.
(c) The eye (episcleritis, less commonly iritis).
(d) Laryngo- or tracheo-broncho-malacia; aortic regurgitation.

160, 161 (a) Early erosive changes at the joint margin, later advanced osteolytic changes with loss of the head of the middle phalanx and splaying of the base of the distal phalanx ('pencil-in-cup' deformity).
(b) Psoriasis.

162–164 (a) Calcification of the intervertebral disc.
(b) Dark pigmentation of the sclera.
(c) Patients with alkaptonuria (homogentisic aciduria) produce urine that darkens on standing. It is associated with homogentisic acid pigment deposition in connective tissue, including sclerae, ear pinnae and hyaline and fibrocartilage (ochronosis), where secondary calcification and degenerative arthropathy results. Urinary and prostatic calculi (dark in colour) may develop, and prostatic calculi can be palpated on rectal examination.
(d) Single-gene recessive autosomal transmission.

165 (a) Polymyalgia rheumatica and multiple myeloma. Multiple myeloma.
(b) Excess plasma cells in bone marrow. Other abnormal investigations include monoclonal paraproteinaemia on immunoelectrophoresis, immunoglobulin light chains (Bence Jones protein) in the urine, raised serum calcium and alkaline phosphatase, elevated ESR, leukaemoid blood film.
(c) Hyperviscosity. Plasmapheresis.
(d) Cyclical chemotherapy including prednisolone, melphalan, cyclophosphamide and vincristine. Radiotherapy to localised bony involvement may alleviate severe pain.

166 (a) Widening of the sacro-iliac joint, with extensive bone destruction.
(b) Tuberculosis.
(c) Initiate with isoniazid (4 mg/kg/24 h p.o.) plus rifampicin (10 mg/kg/24 h p.o.) plus ethambutol (15 mg/kg/24 h p.o.) for 8 weeks. Continue isoniazid with either ethumbatol or rifampicin for 9 months.

167 (a) The appearance of contrast in the left ventricle indicates aortic valve insufficiency.
(b) Mechanical interference with valve function due to granulomatous change and nodule formation contrasts with patchy destruction of the media of the aortic root in ankylosing spondylitis.
(c) Pericardial involvement is much more common than myocardial or endocardial disease. It is usually asymptomatic, but may manifest as chest pain and occasionally lead to tamponade or constrictive (fibrinous) pericarditis. Inflammatory rheumatoid myocarditis is extremely rare.

168 (a) Linear erythema over the dorsum of the fingers, particularly over the PIP and MCP joints. Probable nicotine staining of the right index finger.
(b) Polymyositis/dermatomyositis — CPK, EMG, muscle biopsy. Chest X-ray and any other investigations for malignant disease indicated by the history and examination.
(c) Connective tissue disorder (SLE, scleroderma, mixed connective tissue disease) and malignancy.

169 (a) Erythema marginatum. Rheumatic fever.
(b) Rising anti-streptolysin O-titre, leucocytosis and elevated C reactive protein, first-degree heart block on ECG.
(c) Chorea (Sydenham's).

170 (a) Atlanto-axial subluxation.
(b) Both atlanto-axial subluxation and significant lower cervical vertebral subluxation may result in spinal cord compression, or nerve root traction, causing myelopathy or radiculopathy, or a combination of both.

171, 172 (a) Posterior indentation of 5th vertebral body (long-standing, cortex preserved).
(b) *Cafe-au-lait* spots and dermal nodules indicate neurofibromatosis (von Recklinghausen's disease). Neurofibromata arising from nerve roots may compress spinal canal contents as well as the root itself (the dumbbell tumour).
(c) Scoliosis.

173 (a) Behçet's syndrome. Genital ulceration (painful punched-out scrotal or vulval lesions), erythema nodosum, superficial thrombophlebitis.
(b) Obliterative involvement of blood vessels is a feature of this disease, including large veins (eg inferior vena cava) and arteries, with occasional digital gangrene. Many of the clinical features are believed to have a vasculitic aetiology.
(c) Hypopyon commonly accompanies iritis in this condition. Chronic or recurrent retinal vasculitis may result in blindness.

174 (a) Periosteal reaction along the radial aspect of both 1st metacarpals and the right 2nd metacarpal.
(b) Thyroid acropachy. Exophthalmos, pretibial myxoedema, clubbing, overt hypothyroidism.
(c) High levels of circulating thyroid-stimulating immunoglobulins (eg LATS).

175, 176 (a) Massive soft tissue swelling around 1st MTP joint, with cream-coloured discharge.
(b) Discharging gouty tophus. A tophaceous deposit present at the index DIP joint.
(c) Thiazide diuretics.

177 (a) Patchy, diffuse interstitial lung markings, suggesting diffuse fibrosis.
(b) No. Pulmonary fibrosis is a late manifestation in a few patients with severe rheumatoid disease, and typically is confined to the lower zones.
(c) Non-suppurative granulomata, characteristic of sarcoidosis.
(d) Raised serum calcium and angiotensin converting enzyme. Rheumatoid factor should not be relied on, as it is occasionally present in sarcoidosis.

178, 179 (a) Superimposed joint infection.
(b) Established joint damage, impaired neutrophil chemotaxis and phagocytosis, sepsis of ulcerating skin nodules, increased synovial blood flow, synovial complement consumption with impaired bacterial opsonisation, drug therapy.
(c) Fever, acute single joint inflammation (sepsis is commonly polyarticular at diagnosis) and leukocytosis may all be absent.

180 (a) Joint fusion.
(b) Severe joint disorganisation with loss of femoral head, destruction of acetabular roof, patchy sclerosis and absence of significant osteoporosis. This is a neuropathic joint. Residual opacities from bismuth injection indicate previous treatment of congenital syphilis.

181 (a) Tuberous xanthomata.
(b) Homozygous familial hypercholesterolaemia (WHO-type 2A).
(c) About 20 years.
(d) Obtain measurements of serum cholesterol level and provide appropriate dietary advice.

182 (a) Markedly distended olecranon bursa.
(b) Olecranon bursal swelling of this severity is commonly associated with rheumatoid nodule formation.
(c) In the absence of infection it should usually be left alone. In rheumatoid arthritis control of disease activity may result in improvement. However, a lesion of this size may require surgical excision.

183, 184 (a) Increased isotope uptake most marked at the 11th thoracic vertebra, also at 2nd to 4th lumbar vertebrae. Widening of the body of the 11th thoracic vertebra with preservation of vertebral height and disc space.
(b) Widening of the vertebral body is typical of Paget's disease and may also occur in bone lymphoma. Metastatic disease (eg from breast) should be considered, but the X-ray appearances are not typical.
(c) A markedly raised alkaline phosphatase and 24-h hydroxproline excretion supported the diagnosis of Paget's disease. Careful clinical examination showed no evidence of carcinoma or lymphoma.

185 (a) Livedo reticularis.
(b) Polyarteritis nodosa.
(c) Serious visceral involvement, specifically renal disease (proliferative glomerulitis and necrotising vasculitis), CNS involvement (hemiparesis, cerebellar and brain-stem damage), myocardial involvement (including coronary aneurysm), necrotising damage to gastro-intestinal tract.

(d) Combination high-dose prednisolone and cyclophosphamide. Intermittent pulsing of therapy may improve the benefit: risk ratio.

186 (a) Flattening of the 3rd metatarsal head with sclerosis surrounding a lucent crescent, with preservation of cartilage. Osteonecrosis (osteochondritis dissecans).
(b) Freiberg's infarction.
(c) Early epiphyseal closure (the commonest age is 13–18 years), and late secondary osteoarthrosis.

187 (a) Rubella.
(b) Occipital lymphadenopathy.
(c) Rising titre of rubella antibodies.

188 (a) Osteogenesis imperfecta.
(b) Blue sclerae, thin translucent skin with wide scars, stunting and discolouration of teeth, occasional aortic and/or mitral valve regurgitation.
(c) A variety of defects of collagen synthesis have been demonstrated.

189 (a) Chronic sarcoidosis.
(b) Lupus pernio.
(c) Muscle granulomas may cause localised painful myopathy or muscle nodules, or may be asymptomatic.

190 (a) Increased isotope uptake in bones adjacent to left 2nd and 3rd and right 2nd and 4th MCP joints, left 2nd and 3rd and right 4th and 5th PIP joints, the joints of the left thumb and the left ulnar styloid.
(b) Isotope uptake mirrors increased bone blood flow adjacent to sites of inflammation, and here demonstrated on either side of inflamed joints. The distribution is typical of rheumatoid synovitis.
(c) Any cause of increased bone metabolism such as repair of traumatic, osteoporotic or osteomalacic fractures, Paget's disease, bone destruction by primary or secondary tumour and inflammation within bone (osteomyelitis) or adjacent to bone (penetrating ulcers, soft tissue abscess, joint synovitis or enthesopathy).

191, 192 (a) Swan-neck deformities of all fingers, flexion position of the thumb MP joint.
(b) The only significant abnormality is some MCP ulnar deviation, and mild subluxation of the right thumb MCP joint.
(c) This is an uncommon but well-recognised feature of systemic lupus erythematosus, which this patient has. Hand function remains good.

193 (a) Raynaud's phenomenon.
(b) Progressive systemic sclerosis (and the CREST variant), polymyositis and dermatomyositis, sytemic lupus erythematosus, less commonly rheumatoid arthritis.
(c) Cervical rib and fibrous bands, large-vessel atherosclerosis, occupational vibration trauma, rarely thromboembolism and phaeochromocytoma.

194 (a) Dilation and loop formation in the nail bed capillaries.
(b) Scleroderma. Thickening of the skin of the fingers and the face, with associated telangiectasia. Calcinosis may also be present.
(c) Barium swallow. Loss of oesophageal peristalsis. Endoscopy may be normal or may show reflux oesophagitis.

(d) Increased collagen deposition in the lamina propria and submucosa, particularly in the lower two-thirds of the oesophagus, with muscularis atrophy and mucosal thinning. Small intestinal hypomotility with occasional bacterial overgrowth and malabsorption; wide-mouthed diverticulae, usually on the antimesenteric border of the transverse and descending colon.

195, 196 (a) Increased cartilage thickness with 1st carpometacarpal joint degenerative change.
(b) Acromegaly.
(c) Lateral skull X-ray for pituitary fossa enlargement, and heel pad thickness.
(d) Osteoarthrosis.

197 (a) Scleromalacia.
(b) During healing of scleral damage, collagen fibres laid down in a linear manner remain translucent.

198 (a) Arachnodactyly — Marfan's syndrome.
(b) Dislocation of the lens.
(c) Kyphoscoliosis, anterior chest deformity, pes planus.
(d) Degenerative arthritis at 1st carpo-metacarpal and metacarpo-phalangeal joints.

199 (a) PAS-positive speckled staining within the macrophages.
(b) Whipple's disease.
(c) In addition to fever, hyperpigmentation of exposed areas, peripheral lymphadonopathy and pleural reactions may occur.
(d) The PAS-positive material is associated with rod-shaped organisms infiltrating the lamina propria. Culture of these organisms has not been successful, but treatment with tetracycline (1 g daily for 1 year) results in sustained resolution of arthralgia commencing within 1–4 weeks.

200 (a) Right-axis deviation associated with peaked p-waves (standard lead II); right ventricular hypertrophy with strain. Pulmonary hypertension.
(b) Loud pulmonary second heart sound, sternal or left parasternal heave, pulmonary ejection flow murmur.
(c) Anti-RNP antibody (giving a speckled antinuclear fluorescent staining), usually in high titre.